Medical
Immunology
for Students

QR
42
5

For Churchill Livingstone
Publisher: Timothy Horne
Project Editor: Jim Killgore
Production: Nancy Arnott
Design Direction: Erik Bigland
Sales Promotion Executive: Marion Pollock

Medical Immunology for Students

J. H. L. Playfair MB BChir PhD DSc
Professor and Head, Department of Immunology,
University College London Medical School,
London

P. M. Lydyard BSc MSc PhD
Professor, Department of Immunology,
University College London Medical School,
London

Churchill Livingstone

EDINBURGH LONDON MADRID MELBOURNE NEW YORK AND TOKYO 1995

CHURCHILL LIVINGSTONE
Medical Division of Pearson Professional Ltd

Distributed in the United States of America by
Churchill Livingstone Inc., 650 Avenue of the Americas,
New York, N.Y. 10011, and by associated companies,
branches and representatives throughout the world.

First published 1995
  Reprinted 1995

ISBN 0-443-05000-7

British Library Cataloguing in Publication Data
A catalogue record for this book is available from the British Library.

Library of Congress Cataloging in Publication Data
A catalog record for this book is available from the
Library of Congress.

Produced by Longman Singapore Publishers Pte Ltd
Printed in Singapore

Acknowledgements

We should like to acknowledge the help and advice of all our colleagues in this medical school and elsewhere, including the many students whose constant feedback has, we hope, kept us on the right track. In particular we would like to thank Prof. Peter Beverley, Dr. David Briggs, Prof. Charles Brook, Dr. Jonathan Brostoff, Juliana Chow, Dr. Michael Cole, Dr. Peter Delves, Dr. Pauline Dowd, Jake Eyers, Prof. Carlo Grossi, Prof. David Isenberg, Prof. George Janossy, Prof. David Linch, Prof. Guy Neild, Dr. Michael Shipley, Prof. Howard Thomas, Prof. Mack Turner, Tonia Vincent, Dr. David Webster, Prof. Ian Weller and Dr. Alex Whelan, who kindly looked at early drafts. Any residual errors are our own, not theirs. We also owe, of course, an enormous debt to the authors of the longer textbooks which we regularly use and which are mentioned in the *reading list*.

We also gratefully acknowledge permission for use of the following illustrations:

- Page 6 Figs 1a & 1b From Roitt I M, Brostoff J, Male D 1989 Immunology, 2nd edn. Gower Medical Publishing, London: Fig. 2.33, p. 2.15 and Fig. 2.27, p. 2.2
- Page 6 Fig. 1c From Stevens A, Lowe J 1992 Histology. Gower Medical Publishing, London: Fig. 11.3, p. 178
- Page 6 Fig. 3a From Immunology (Gower Medical): Fig. 2.35, p. 2.15
- Page 6 Fig. 3b From Burkitt H G, Young B, Heath J W, 1993 Wheater's functional histology, 3rd edn. Churchill Livingstone, Edinburgh: Fig. 1.4c, p. 8
- Page 6 Fig. 3c From Austin Gresham G 1971 A colour atlas of general pathology. Wolfe Publishing, London: Fig. 153, p. 134
- Page 8 Fig. 3a & 3b From Schaechter M, Medhoff G, Schlessinger D 1989 Mechanisms of microbial disease. Williams and Wilkins, Baltimore: Fig. 4.8, p. 83 and Fig. 4.7, p. 83
- Page 10 Fig. 1 With permission of Prof. M. B. Pepys and Dr. E. A. Munn
- Page 12 Fig. 2 From Immunology (Gower Medical): Fig. 2.17, p. 2.8
- Page 16 Fig. 1a From Wheater's functional histology (Churchill Livingstone): Fig. 3.8, p. 51
- Page 16 Fig. 1b From Roitt I M 1991 Essential immunology, 7th edn. Blackwell Scientific, Oxford: Fig. 2.7a, p. 22
- Page 18 Fig. 3a From Immunology (Gower Medical): Fig. 2.22, p. 2.10
- Page 18 Fig. 3b With permission of Prof. C. E. Grossi
- Page 24 Fig. 2b From Essential immunology (Blackwell Scientific): Fig. 3.16b, p. 49
- Page 38 Fig. 2 From Madeley C R, Field A M, 1988 Virus morphology, 2nd edn. Churchill Livingstone, Edinburgh: Plate 30, p. 86
- Page 38 Fig. 4 With permission of Dr. J. Holton
- Page 38 Fig. 5 With permission of Dr. S. Lucas
- Page 38 Figs 6 & 7 From Peters W, Gilles H M, 1977 A colour atlas of tropical medicine and parasitology. Wolfe Medical Publications, London: Fig. 125, p. 67 and Fig. 331, p. 172
- Page 44 Figs 1 & 2 From A colour atlas of general pathology (Wolfe Publishing): Fig. 200, p. 169 and Fig. 198, p. 167
- Page 44 Fig. 3 From More I A R, Brown I L, 1994 Colour guide general pathology. Churchill Livingstone, Edinburgh: Fig. 45, p. 30
- Page 44 Figs 4, 5 & 6 With permission of Dr. S. Lucas
- Page 62 Fig. 1a From Brostoff J, Scadding G K, Male D, Roitt I M (eds) 1991 Clinical immunology. Gower Medical Publishing, London: Fig. 6.26, p. 6.13
- Page 62 Fig. 1b Reproduced by permission of Edward Arnold (Publishers) Ltd. From Anderson J R (ed) 1976 Muir's textbook of pathology. Edward Arnold, London: Fig. 18.20, p. 547
- Page 62 Fig. 1c From Clinical immunology (Gower Medical): Fig. 10.8, p. 10.4
- Page 62 Figs 1d & 1e With permission of Dr S. Lucas.
- Page 62 Fig. 1f Reproduced by permission of Edward Arnold (Publishers) Ltd. From Muir's textbook of pathology (Edward Arnold): Fig. 19.30, p. 626
- Page 66 Fig. 1a, 1b & 1c With permission of Dr. M. Griffiths
- Page 68, Fig. 4 From Souhami R L, Moxham J (eds) 1994 Textbook of Medicine, 2nd edn. Churchill Livingstone, Edinburgh: Fig. 22.40, p. 959
- Page 72 Figs 3 & 4 From Clinical immunology (Gower Medical): Fig. 5.4, p. 5.2 and Fig. 5.6, p. 5.3
- Page 74 Fig. 1 With permission of Prof. D. Isenberg
- Page 92 Fig. 1 With permission of Prof. A. Segal and Dr. M. Smith.

London   J. H. L. P.
1995   P. M. L.

Introduction

Immunology is mainly to do with infection

In medicine and related subjects, we study the normal working of the body and its systems, the diseases that affect it and their treatment. Underlying much of medicine is the concept that the body has ways of **resisting** and recovering from disease. In the important case of infectious disease, these resistance mechanisms are collectively called immunity, and the study of this is termed **immunology.** In fact, the scope of immunology is wider than just defence against infection, because when immune mechanisms malfunction, as quite often happens, they themselves can cause disease — usually referred to as **immunopathology**.

Immunology can be both basic and clinical

In this book, we consider Immunology under three main headings, which correspond to the parts of the undergraduate courses in which most students encounter the subject.

1. First we look at the normal workings of the immune system, which are usually taught alongside other aspects of physiology, biochemistry, genetics, etc. early in the curriculum; this might conveniently be termed **basic immunology** and the student will find frequent cross-referencing to other topics usually encountered by both medical and science students.

2. Next we turn to those aspects of immunology touching on mechanisms of disease, which are generally taught as part of the **pathology** course, emphasizing their links with histopathology, chemical pathology, and microbiology.

3. Finally we review the **clinical conditions** in which immunological processes play a part or may need to be assessed. In line with the usual layout of the clinical curriculum, these are considered by system so that the medical student can refer to the relevant section while proceeding through the medical and surgical firms. We hope this section will also be of value to students of dentistry, nursing, podiatry, etc. who will come into contact with patients.

Adapting this book to your course

We realise that this may not be the sequence followed in all curricula, but we hope that the book's layout, in which each double-page spread corresponds to a 50-minute lecture, will allow students to take topics in a different order where appropriate; the clinical sections, for example, would obviously not always be taught in the same sequence. As presented, the course is one that has evolved over many years in the medical and science schools of the Middlesex Hospital and University College London, and we believe it works well, emphasizing that immunology is not a small esoteric speciality but a discipline that permeates almost the whole of medicine and biology. It should be emphasized that we have included only those parts of the subject that we feel the student really needs; there is of course an enormous amount more, and those with the timeand courage to tackle this should start by consulting the reading lists given on the first four *tutorial pages* and p.57. We hope these tutorials will also be found useful for self-assessment at each stage of the course. Technical details that we felt the student should know about will found in the *appendix*.

London
1995

J. H. L. P.
P. M. L.

Contents

Basic Immunology

Immunopathology

Clinical Immunology

Investigating the Immune System

Appendices

Index

Defence Mechanisms (1)

External defences

Strictly speaking, defence against infectious organisms starts with the outer coatings of the body which, if intact, function as *barriers* to invasion. These include the skin and mucous membranes together with their various glands and secretions (Fig. 1). Though these are not normally considered as immunological, the distinction is rather artificial and their role in keeping out infection is extremely important. In later sections we shall see the results of defects in the microbicidal activity of the skin. We shall also discuss the interesting question of why certain microorganisms attempt to enter the body while others remain on the outside and whether entry is always harmful to the host. You will see that *infection* is not always synonymous with *disease*.

Internal defences

Infectious organisms that do gain entry encounter an impressive array of internal defence mechanisms and this is where immunology really comes in. Essentially, what is needed is to *recognize* the invaders and *dispose* of them. Some recognition and disposal mechanisms are already present, rather like policemen patrolling the streets, while others can be mobilized into action within a few minutes or hours. Others take longer still — days or weeks. The early defence mechanisms are conventionally lumped together under the title of **natural immunity**.

Natural immunity: the rapid defence system

This includes a variety of cells and molecules whose presence can be literally life-saving; we shall see just how important they are when we consider conditions in which they are deficient. There is, however, a price to be paid for such rapid activity, which is that it is fairly vague in its aim. Indeed in the early stages of infection, the precise target may not yet have been identified beyond the recognition that it is, for example, probably a virus or a bacterium. Thus, in police terms, natural immunity responds somewhat on the 'round up all the usual suspects' principle. In immunological jargon, this lack of precision is referred to as **non-specific**, by contrast with the very high specificity of later responses (p. 3) but, as will be seen, specificity is relative and a better term for natural immunity might be 'low specificity'. Another name sometimes used is **innate**, which reflects the fact that most natural immune mechanisms are present at birth, and indeed before it, and do not change greatly with age. Thus natural, non-specific and innate immunity all mean essentially the same thing.

The importance of the macrophage

The main cells and molecules responsible for natural immunity are shown in Figure 2, in which the central role of the **macrophage** is emphasized. Indeed, macrophages are probably the single most important cell type in immunity and a complete absence of macrophages would almost certainly be incompatible with survival. Together with the **polymorphonuclear (PMN) neutrophils** they are responsible for recognizing and removing unwanted particulate matter, a process known as **phagocytosis** (see p. 6); they secrete a huge variety of molecules including the anti-viral **interferon**, the anti-bacterial **lysozyme** and other molecules that stimulate the liver to release **acute phase proteins**, valuable in limiting both tissue damage and infection. Macrophages and liver cells also keep up the level of **complement**, which helps in several ways to dispose of bacteria. Complement and **mast cells** interact to increase blood flow and vascular permeability, which leads to the signs of **inflammation**. Another type of cell, the **natural killer (NK) cell**, which is part of the early response to virus infection, is also considered as belonging to the natural immune system since it shows the same characteristic features of rapid action and low specificity.

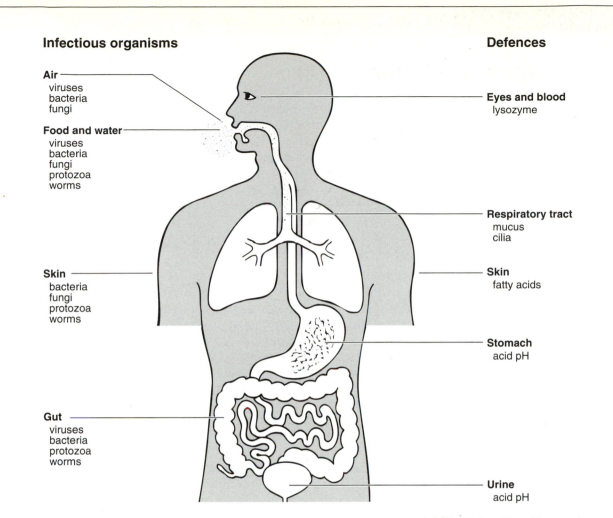

Infectious organisms

Air
viruses
bacteria
fungi

Food and water
viruses
bacteria
fungi
protozoa
worms

Skin
bacteria
fungi
protozoa
worms

Gut
viruses
bacteria
protozoa
worms

Defences

Eyes and blood
lysozyme

Respiratory tract
mucus
cilia

Skin
fatty acids

Stomach
acid pH

Urine
acid pH

Fig. 1 The external defences of the body. The air we breathe, our skin and our intestinal tract are crowded with microbes. Most of these are bacteria and viruses, with occasional fungi, but in tropical countries protozoa and helminths (worms) add further to the burden. Bactericidal skin secretions, gastric acidity, and mucus and cilia in the bronchial tree help to reduce the load while intact epithelium generally keeps them from entering the tissues. In the blood and secretions, the enzyme lysozyme kills many bacteria by attacking their cell walls. IgA antibody (see p.23) is also important in the defence of mucous surfaces.

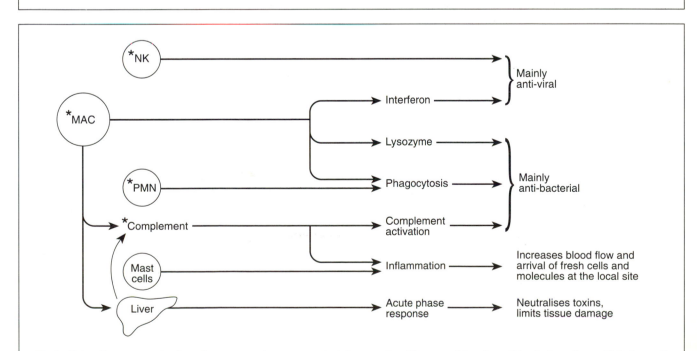

Fig. 2 Natural immune mechanisms form a general purpose, early defence system. They come into action within minutes or hours of infection and/ or tissue damage. Note that all these components are relatively non-specific in terms of both recognition and disposal, but some (*) do have the ability to recognize foreign material. However, unlike adaptive mechanisms (p. 3), they do not retain any memory of their encounter with infectious organisms but simply return to 'baseline'. NK, natural killer cells; MAC, macrophage; PMN, polymorphonuclear leucocyte (neutrophil).

Defence Mechanisms (2)

In almost all cases, one or other of the elements of the natural immune system will successfully deal with the threat of infection. Bacteria may be phagocytosed by macrophages or PMN, perhaps with the help of complement; virus replication may be halted by interferon or the virus-infected cells killed by NK cells; the inflammatory response will ensure a good supply of fresh cells and molecules via the blood stream; acute phase proteins will limit damage and mop up toxins. In fact the great majority of animals rely on defence of this sort because, until the evolution of the vertebrates, this was all they had – and invertebrates can hardly be called unsuccessful in surviving!

Adaptive immunity: a new form of defence

Nevertheless, just before the first sharks and fishes appeared, at the beginning of vertebrate evolution, nature seems to have felt the need for something more in the way of defence against infection. What she came up with was a quite amazing new system within which the ability to *recognize* particular invading microbes was enormously expanded, to the point where — again in police terms — there was virtually one policeman allocated to each criminal. This required some very complex gene duplications and rearrangements and a new type of cell, the **lymphocyte**. From now on, animals could mount immune responses in which the disposal mechanisms were focused on the precise microbe in question, like marksmen shooting at an identified target rather than wildly in all directions; in immunological language the recognition was highly **specific**. Some of the lymphocytes also carried out the destruction and disposal themselves but others released molecules called **antibody** which homed in on the target and marked it for destruction by the disposal mechanisms of natural immunity: macrophages, complement, etc. (Fig. 1). The genes coding for these new recognition molecules can generate new mutations and combinations with unusual rapidity, so the ones that lead to survival will be strongly selected for during evolution. Thus, the species, and even the individual, can gradually adapt towards responding optimally to those infections it repeatedly meets. For this reason, the whole lymphocyte-based system is known as **adaptive immunity**; the terms specific and acquired are sometimes used to convey the same idea, but in this book we shall refer to it throughout as adaptive.

Advantages and disadvantages

This tremendous improvement in specificity made it extremely difficult for any infectious microorganisms to escape being recognized, though many of them learned how to avoid destruction, as indeed they must in order to survive at all. However, there was a price to pay for the improved specificity of adaptive immunity in that lymphocytes require considerably more time to carry out their functions than macrophages, mast cells, etc. so that an adaptive immune response may take days or even weeks to become effective. This inherent *slowness* is one of the drawbacks of adaptive immunity, but here too the lymphocyte shows its extraordinary potential, thanks to the development of **memory**, which allows all subsequent responses to the same infection to proceed much more rapidly. Thus a **'secondary' adaptive response** can be almost as rapid as a natural immune response. Specificity and memory are the hallmarks of adaptive immunity and they always imply that lymphocytes are involved. An everyday example of the adaptive system in action is the 'immunity' that follows an attack of measles (Fig. 2); people who have had the disease before produce antibody so fast that the virus is eliminated before it can cause symptoms, whereas during the first infection you can be ill for a week or more while the lymphocytes go about their preliminary work. By contrast, if natural immunity had been able to cope with the measles virus, you would not have been ill even the first time. One other potential drawback of adaptive immunity is that it can more easily go wrong and injure the host (the field of **immunopathology**). In later sections we shall study in detail how all this operates.

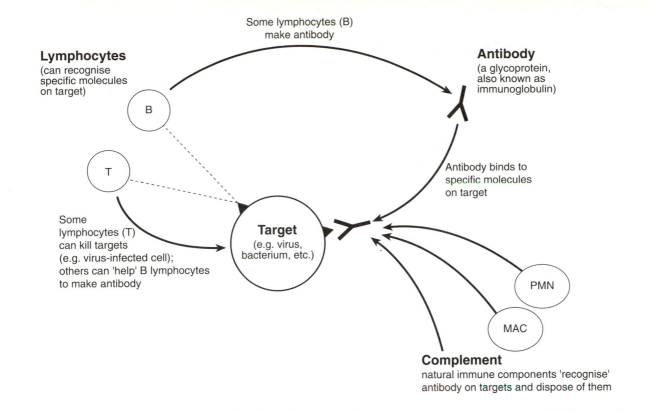

Fig. 1 Adaptive immunity is based on the activities of lymphocytes. Each of these cells can specifically recognize one out of the thousands of molecular shapes found on infectious organisms — the 'targets' of the immune system. One type of lymphocyte, known as B, then makes antibody, which binds to the same molecule that induced it, marking the target for disposal by natural immune elements. Another type, known as T, can do many things including killing some targets but also helping other cells to function properly.

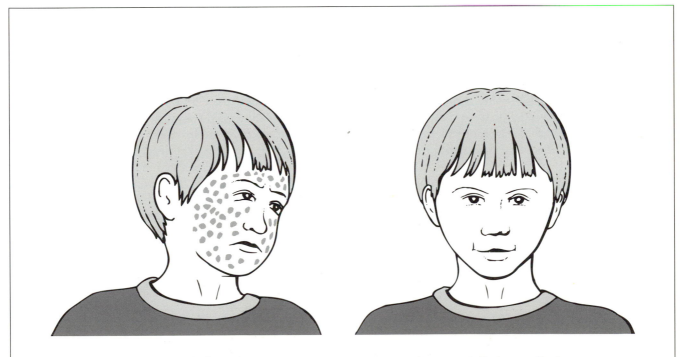

In a first attack of measles, adaptive immunity is too slow to prevent the virus growing and causing symptoms

In a second attack, an antibody response is made so rapidly that the virus is disposed of before symptoms appear

Fig. 2 Measles and other common childhood infections illustrate the ability of the adaptive immune system to 'learn' from previous experience. In many cases a harmless vaccine can be used to induce this 'memory' without the need to suffer the primary infection.

Phagocytosis

The most ancient defence system

Water, ions and molecules must pass into and out of all living cells and the various mechanisms of **endocytosis** and **exocytosis** are covered in cell biology textbooks. A specialized form of endocytosis occurs in certain cells as part of the disposal of outdated body components such as denatured proteins, aged red cells, products of tissue damage, etc. and it makes use of a very similar process to that by which free-living protozoa ingest their food, namely **phagocytosis**. This is of great importance in immunology because the same cells are also responsible for taking in and destroying foreign particulate matter, including microorganisms. Even in higher vertebrates, possessing very complex and refined immune systems, phagocytosis is still a major part of the defence against infection, though for its proper functioning it often needs help from other elements such as antibody and complement, as described in later sections.

Two kinds of phagocyte

There are two main populations of phagocytic cells:

- mononuclear **macrophages**
- polymorphonuclear **neutrophils**.

In this book we shall refer to the latter as PMN (Fig. 1). Both are produced in the bone marrow, the former circulating for about 24 hours as **monocytes** before settling in the tissues as macrophages, where they may live for months or years. The shorter-lived (4–5 days) PMN circulate in the blood unless attracted into the tissues to deal with an acute infection, especially by bacteria or fungi. The characteristic pus of a bacterial abscess is composed largely of decomposed PMN. Macrophages are found in most organs, especially the liver, lungs, spleen and bone marrow; the liver contains about 90% of the total body population in the form of the Kupffer cells that line the sinusoids. The role of macrophages in the control of chronic infection and in chronic inflammation will be discussed later.

A multi-step event

The process of phagocytosis is essentially the same in PMN and macrophages and can usefully be divided into six stages (Figs 2 & 3). First the cell must *move* to where it is needed, which often involves following **chemotactic** gradients of microbial or immunological molecules. Next the particle to be phagocytosed must *attach* to the cell; this may occur because cell surface molecules *recognize* surface molecules on the microbe (these are mainly protein–sugar interactions), but it may also be complement or antibody that is recognized, by corresponding receptors on the phagocyte. This is known as **opsonization**. Membrane movements, involving the cytoskeleton, then lead to the particle being *internalized* — taken into an intracellular vesicle called a **phagosome**. This then normally *fuses* with a number of vesicles called **lysosomes** that contain microbicidal components such as oxygen free radicals and various toxic proteins (p. 35), which are able to *kill* the majority of bacteria, fungi, etc. They also contain a variety of digestive enzymes which break down the dead microbe into small molecular components that can be reutilized or, in other words, *dispose* of it.

A two-way battle

The above is the ideal scenario (from the host's point of view!) but it does not always go so smoothly. The phagocytes may be defective at one stage or another; PMN are particularly susceptible to genetic abnormalities (p. 53). Or the microbe may take evasive action, for example by resisting internalization or killing, as will be discussed in a later section (pp. 37–40). Sometimes they can be killed but not completely digested, which can lead to chronic inflammation. Therefore, it is best to think of the encounter between microbe and phagocyte as a two-way battle, from which sometimes one side emerges victorious and sometimes the other.

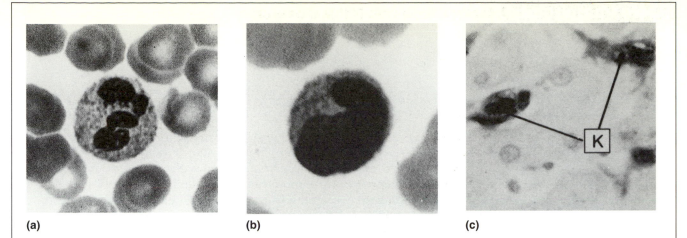

Fig. 1 The principal phagocytic cells. (a) PMN in blood; (b) monocyte in blood; (c) macrophages in tissue (Kuppfer cells in the liver).

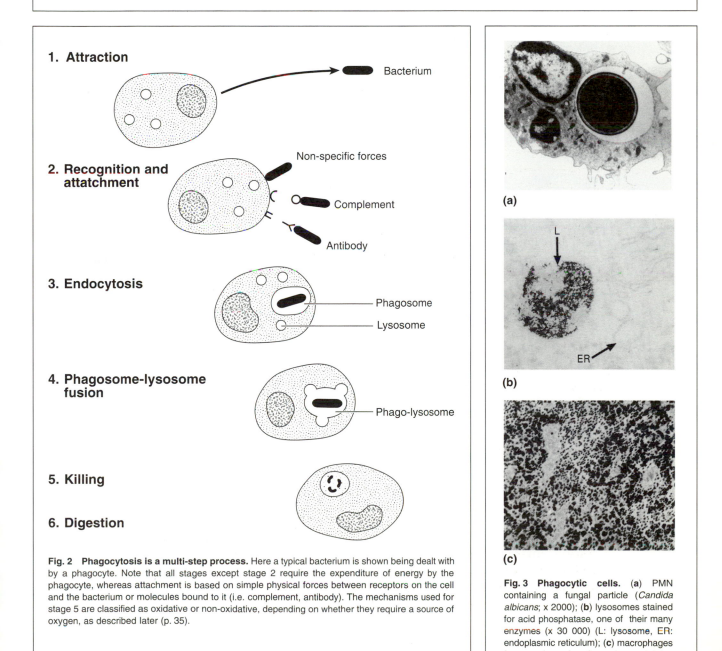

1. Attraction

Bacterium

2. Recognition and attatchment

Non-specific forces

Complement

Antibody

3. Endocytosis

Phagosome

Lysosome

4. Phagosome-lysosome fusion

Phago-lysosome

5. Killing

6. Digestion

Fig. 2 Phagocytosis is a multi-step process. Here a typical bacterium is shown being dealt with by a phagocyte. Note that all stages except stage 2 require the expenditure of energy by the phagocyte, whereas attachment is based on simple physical forces between receptors on the cell and the bacterium or molecules bound to it (i.e. complement, antibody). The mechanisms used for stage 5 are classified as oxidative or non-oxidative, depending on whether they require a source of oxygen, as described later (p. 35).

(a)

L

ER

(b)

(c)

Fig. 3 Phagocytic cells. (a) PMN containing a fungal particle (*Candida albicans*; x 2000); (b) lysosomes stained for acid phosphatase, one of their many enzymes (x 30 000) (L: lysosome, ER: endoplasmic reticulum); (c) macrophages from a lung lymph node containing inhaled coal dust. Not only microbes are removed by these useful cells (x 30).

6

Complement

A cascade system

Four 'cascade' systems of molecules are present in the plasma, waiting to respond to tissue damage and induce inflammation. Of these, the **complement** system is the most important in relation to infection, although its effects do overlap to some extent with the other three (the clotting, fibrinolytic and kinin systems, whose main roles are in tissue repair). It is also the most complex, consisting of about 20 proteins, capable of being activated in two distinct ways and leading to three different useful results (Fig. 1). Its strange name was invented 100 years ago on account of just one of its properties – that of helping antibody dispose of bacteria.

The central component: C 3

Rather than trying to memorize the names, molecular weights, cleavage products and components shown in Figure 2 (which the doctor does *not* need to know by heart!), it is better to picture one of them, known as the '3rd component' or **C3**, as the heart of the system. C3 is a major serum protein (about 1 g/litre) whose enzymatic splitting or *activation* has dramatic effects. If it occurs on the surface of a bacterial cell, most of the C3 is left there (it is now known as C3b) and it marks the bacterium out for phagocytosis because phagocytic cells have receptors that recognize and attach to C3b. In such a case, the bacterium is said to be opsonized. C3b also acts as a focus for other complement components (C5, C6, C7, C8, C9) to collect and form into small pores that puncture the cell membrane and make it leak and eventually die — a process known as lysis (Fig. 3). Opsonization and (to a lesser extent) **lysis** are responsible for the destruction of many bacterial and fungal cells.

Inflammation

The small piece cleaved off C3, which is known as C3a, has a completely different function. Together with C5a (derived in the same way from C5), it promotes **inflammation** by attracting and activating PMN and mast cells, with the result that local vascular permeability increases and PMN, monocytes, antibodies and more complement, etc. flow into the tissues. C3a and C5a are known as **anaphylatoxins**. Inflammation will feature later in the book (e.g. pp. 11 & 43).

Two pathways of activation

This all-important cleavage of C3 can be caused in two ways (Fig. 1). It may occur spontaneously on the surface of cells such as bacteria, with help from factors B and D and properdin (the system has ingenious inhibitors to stop it happening on the body's own cells); this is called the **alternative pathway** of complement activation because it was only discovered recently; but in evolutionary terms it was probably the earliest. The other, known as the **classical pathway**, requires the presence of antibody. It involves a sequence of steps starting with the binding of C1q, C1r, and C1s to antibody molecules that have come together by binding to the same foreign particle and the subsequent activation of C4 and C2 to form an enzyme or convertase that can cleave C3. Thus, wherever antibody molecules are bound to, for example, a bacterium, there will now be C3b as well, and since phagocytic cells can recognize both C3b and antibody molecules (again via receptors), the chances that the bacterium will end up inside the phagocyte are tremendously increased (Fig. 4). Indeed the combination of phagocytic cells, complement and antibody represents the most formidable obstacle to the survival of bacteria and fungi and a deficiency of any one of these three elements can result in serious recurrent infections.

Receptors for complement are found not only on phagocytes but also on red cells and on B lymphocytes (the Epstein–Barr virus uses a complement receptor to attach to these cells and infect them, causing glandular fever). In later sections we describe other links between complement and disease, including the ways in which complement activation can occur inappropriately or get out of control, leading to pathology.

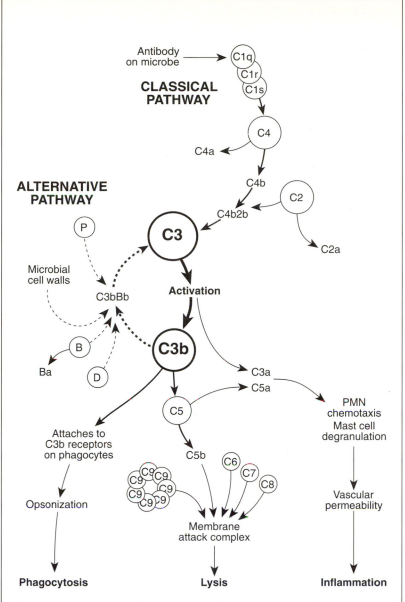

CLASSICAL PATHWAY

Antibody on microbe → C1q C1r C1s

ALTERNATIVE PATHWAY

C4 → C4a
C4b
C4b2b → **C3** ← C2 → C2a

P
Microbial cell walls
C3bBb → **Activation**

B → Ba
D

C3b
Attaches to C3b receptors on phagocytes
C5 → C5a
C3a → PMN chemotaxis
Mast cell degranulation

Opsonization
C5b C6 C7 C8
C9 C9 C9 C9 C9 C9 C9 C9
Membrane attack complex

Vascular permeability

Phagocytosis · **Lysis** · **Inflammation**

Fig. 1 Complement activation, emphasizing the central role of C3. Top: the classical pathway, involving antibody. Centre left: the alternative pathway, which 'ticks over' slowly and is accelerated when it occurs on the surface of, for example, a bacterium. Lower half: the three biological effects of complement — phagocytosis, lysis and inflammation.

Component	Molecular weight (kDa)	Serum level (µg/ml)	Function
C1q	400	250	Classical pathway
C1r	170	100	
C1s	80	80	
C4	210	430	
C2	120	20	
B	100	150	Alternative pathway
D	25	2	
P	220	30	
C3	190	1300	Lytic pathway
C5	180	75	
C6	150	60	
C7	140	60	
C8	150	80	
C9	80	50	
C1 inh	105	180	Inhibitors
C4 b–p	70 (x6)	250	
I		50	
H	155	300	
DAF		150	
CR1	200		Receptors
CR2	140		
CR3	260		

Fig. 2 The principal proteins of the complement pathway. B, D, factors B and D; P, properdin, an enhancing factor for the alternative pathway; DAF, decay accelerating factor; C1 inh, C1 inhibitor; C4 b–p, C4 binding protein. These inhibitors, with factors H and I, restrict the effects of activated C1, C3 and/or C4. CR1, the complement receptor on red cells, does this too, as well as transporting antigen–antibody complexes to the liver macrophages. The other CRs are on the phagocytes themselves.

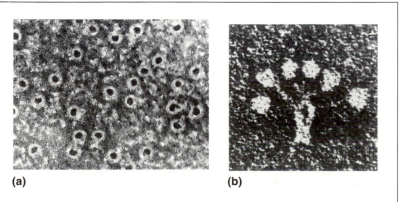

(a) (b)

Fig. 3 Complement under the electron microscope. (a) Holes in the wall of a bacterium made by the membrane attack complex C5–9; (b) the C1q molecule, which interacts with antibody to initiate the classical pathway.

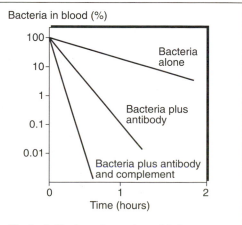

Bacteria in blood (%)

Bacteria alone
Bacteria plus antibody
Bacteria plus antibody and complement

Time (hours)

Fig. 4 Antibody and complement help remove bacteria from blood. Injected bacteria are removed from the blood more rapidly in the presence of antibody, but removal can be even further accelerated by complement.

The Acute Phase Response/Interferon

Acute phase response

Emergency measures

Early after infection and/or injury, a number of the body's homeostatic systems are 're-set' to cope with the changed conditions. These include temperature, nitrogen balance and fat turnover, but also the serum level of certain proteins. Some, such as albumin, fall. Others rise, sometimes dramatically, and these, known as **acute phase proteins**, mostly seem to be involved in either damage limitation (e.g. proteolytic enzyme inhibitors, coagulation factors) or the attempt to reduce bacterial toxicity. Of those in the second category, the best known is **C-reactive protein** (Fig. 1), a pentameric molecule that binds to bacterial phospholipids, activates complement and promotes phagocytosis. In other words it behaves rather like an antibody of very restricted specificity. Its level can rise 1000-fold in a few hours, and it is often used by clinicians to monitor inflammatory diseases. **Fibrinogen** too can rise, which is the basis of the increase in erythrocyte sedimentation rate (ESR), known to the ancient Greeks. Several other acute phase proteins also bind bacterial products, such as toxins, though it must be admitted that their functions are not all understood. A list of the generally accepted acute phase proteins is given in Figure 2.

The macrophage again!

The acute phase proteins are made in liver cells, but the stimulus to their increased production comes from the macrophage, in the form of secreted proteins called **cytokines**, which will be discussed in a later section (p. 33). Cytokines are also responsible for fever and some of the other changes mentioned above, emphasizing once again the extraordinarily important role of macrophages in defence.

Interferon

Early defence against viruses

The name **interferon** (**IFN** for short) refers to a family of proteins made by various cells following viral infection that have the ability to stop virus growth in other cells. Three members of the family are recognized, and the nomenclature is rather confusing. IFNα and IFNβ are very similar molecules produced in macrophages, fibroblasts, etc. early after virus infection and can be considered as part of natural immunity. IFNγ, on the other hand, is structurally different and is made by (T) lymphocytes as part of their adaptive immune response and by NK cells, and has many properties besides being anti-viral (see Cytokines, p.33). If this had been understood when the interferons were discovered (in the 1950s) the nomenclature would probably have been different. Some older names, together with details of the molecules, are shown in Figure 3.

A non-specific anti-viral agent

All known viruses induce IFN, and so do many other microbes. IFN is also active against all viruses, though not always to the same extent. Figure 4 summarizes how it works, the key target being viral RNA translation into protein; however, it is not fully understood why the cell's own protein synthesis is not inhibited too. IFNα is especially interesting to the medical profession because it was one of the first molecules to be purified and used experimentally as therapy — not only for virus infections but also for cancer. Nowadays it is available in genetically engineered form and has an established place in the treatment of certain infections and tumours.

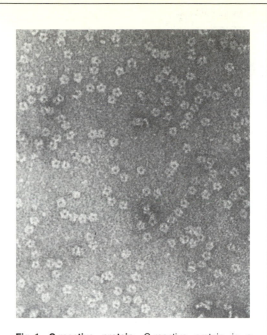

Fig. 1 C-reactive protein. C-reactive protein is a pentameric molecule of molecular weight 120 kDa (i.e. larger than albumin but smaller than antibody). It has been conserved through evolution and a similar molecule is found in crabs. It binds strongly to phosphoryl choline, a component of many bacterial cell walls.

Factor of increase	Protein	Function
x 1000	*C-Reactive protein	Anti-bacterial ?
	*Serum amyloid precursor	?
x 2–4	α_1 anti-trypsin	
	α_1 anti-chymotrypsin }	Protease inhibition
	*α_1 acid glycoprotein	Transport
	Fibrinogen	Coagulation
	Haptoglobin	Haemoglobin binding
+ 50%	*Complement C3, C4	Anti-bacterial inflammatory
	Caeruloplasmin	Scavenges oxygen radicals
	Fibronectin	
	Angiotensinogen	Raises blood pressure
	Mannose-binding protein	? Anti-bacterial
Fall	Albumin, transferrin	

Fig. 2 Acute phase proteins. These are usually classified according to the degree to which they increase during the response. For most of them, a cytokine called IL-6 is the stimulus, but some (*) also require IL-1.

	IFNα	IFNβ	IFNγ
Number of genes	> 20	1	1
Chromosome		9	12
Molecular weight		23 000	15–25 000
Evolution	All vertebrates except amphibia		Mammals only?
Cell origin	All cells, especially macrophages, fibroblasts		T cells, NK cells
Induced by	Mainly viruses; also some bacteria, protozoa; also cytokines		Recognition of antigen by T-cell receptor
Functions	Mainly anti-viral; increase MHC I expression; anti-proliferative		Anti-viral; increase MHC II expression; activate macrophages
Other names	Macrophage; fibroblast Type I		Immune Type II

Fig. 3 The interferon family. Note the similarities between IFNβ and the various IFNαs, which only differ slightly in their anti-viral and anti-proliferative effects. IFNγ is a quite different molecule, interacting with a different receptor, and with widespread effects on immune cells and responses (see p. 33).

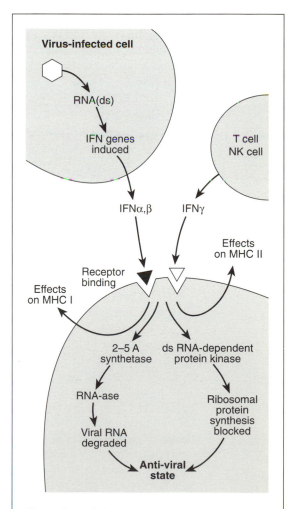

Fig. 4 The anti-viral effect of IFN. This is mainly on viral RNA and its translation into protein, but there may also be some effect on viral entry into cells, transcription and assembly. Note that IFNγ binds to a different receptor from IFNα and β. ds, double-stranded.

Mast Cells and Inflammation/Natural Killer Cells

Inflammation

How inflammation starts

Throughout the connective tissue and particularly in the skin, the lung and the intestine is a population of cells which are extremely sensitive to injury. When damaged by trauma, heat, toxins, etc. they release the contents of their granules (degranulate) and help to initiate the **acute inflammatory response**. These are the **mast cells**, and their granules contain large amounts of **histamine** and other molecules that act on blood vessels. As a result, blood flow is increased and the processes of damage-limitation and control of infection begin. Mast cells also respond to stimuli from complement components (C3a, C5a), from PMN-derived enzymes and from certain kinds of antibody (IgE; p. 23), so that they are quite intimately bound up with both natural and adaptive immunity. The same is true for the blood **basophils**, which are similar in many respects to mast cells.

Unpleasant but useful

A typical example of an acute inflammatory response would be the red, warm, painful swelling of a finger burned or infected with staphylococci. Though unpleasant, it is a sign that useful processes are at work and quite often the growth and spread of bacteria is more rapid and dangerous if inflammation is absent. Sometimes, of course, the presence of an inflammatory response can itself be dangerous, e.g. if it occurs in a limited area such as the airways or the brain, or if it leads to breakdown of vital tissue, e.g. a burst appendix. Sometimes, for various reasons, inflammation becomes *chronic*, and then we are in the realm of **pathology**, which is dealt with in a later section. But it should be remembered that inflammatory responses nearly always start with a good intention: that of limiting tissue damage, restricting infection and initiating repair (Fig. 1).

Natural killer cells

When a lymphocyte is not a lymphocyte

The well-known lymphocytes found in the blood and lymphoid organs are clearly the key cells of adaptive immunity, as will be described in the following sections. They have the required properties of high specificity and memory. However there is another population of cells in the blood which, though they look like lymphocytes, behave differently in that they can kill certain other types of cell without any evidence of specificity or memory. Often referred to as **large granular lymphocytes** because of their appearance (Fig. 2), they are nowadays referred to as **natural killer cells** (NK for short).

A different recognition system

The exact role of NK cells in immunity is hard to judge. In many ways they behave like lymphocytes (the T subset) in that they can kill virus-infected cells and some tumour cells, and also produce the cytokines that are so important in cell–cell communication (p. 33). In other words their **effector** mechanisms (this is immunological jargon for 'what they do') are similar to those of T lymphocytes. But the way they *recognize* their target is quite different — indeed they seem to be best at recognizing just those types of target that T lymphocytes do not. For instance, they do not bind to MHC molecules (p. 19). Another difference is that they act rapidly and do not need to build up their numbers slowly as T lymphocytes do, which is why they are considered as part of the natural immune system (Fig. 3).

From the medical point of view, their main effect is probably in virus infection, because when they are deficient it is viral disease that the patient suffers from. The fact that total absence of NK cells is very rare suggests they do have an important function, though this argument is never 100% watertight.

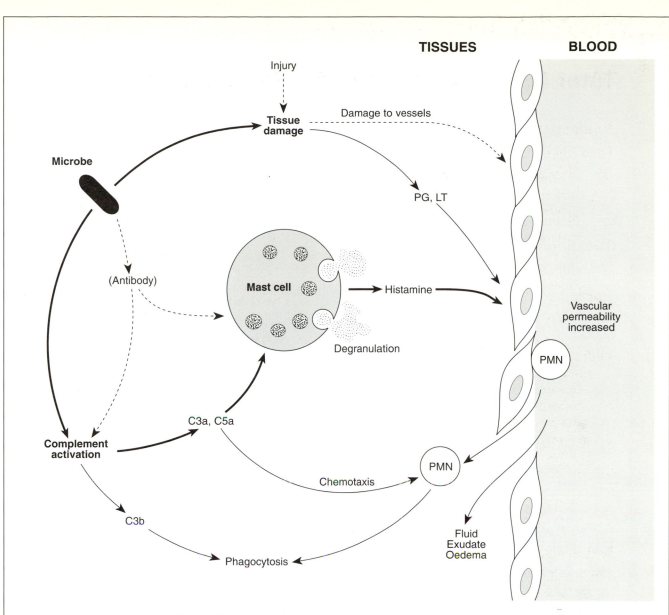

Fig. 1   Inflammatory response in infection. This simplified scheme emphasizes those aspects of acute inflammation of particular relevance to defence against infection. You will hear plenty more about inflammation in your pathology course, where the non-infectious causes, such as injury, burning, etc. will be brought out. PG: prostaglandins; LT: leukotrienes; these are both products of arachidonic acid from cell membranes and, together with histamine and other mast cell products, are the main chemical basis of inflammation.

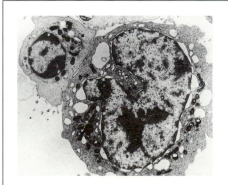

Fig. 2   Natural killer cell. A large granular lymphocyte (NK cell; top left) bound to a tumour cell which is in the process of dying. NK cells also kill non-malignant cells infected with viruses.

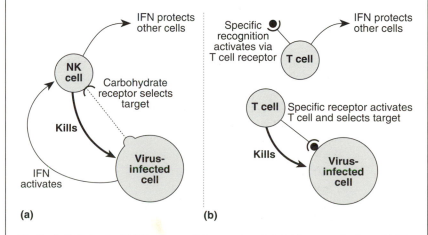

Fig. 3   Anti-viral cells. (a) NK cells constitute an early anti-viral defence mechanism, which is later taken over by **(b)** the slower but more specific and multi-functional T cells (see later sections for more on T cells, including how they recognize their targets). This is a good example of Natural and Adaptive immunity achieving similar results by different means — the main difference here being at the recognition stage.

Tutorial 1

At this point you should have a clear concept of natural immunity and how it works. Before proceeding to the next sections on adaptive immunity, you should attempt to answer (briefly!) the following questions. Compare your answers with the versions on the opposite page and, if you were seriously out, go back and read the relevant section again. No student is expected to *know* everything, but if there is something you do not *understand*, it would be pointless to go further until you have sorted it out.

Questions

Cover up the answers opposite until you have made your attempt.

1. Name three features that distinguish natural and adaptive immune mechanisms.

2. Name three ways in which macrophages contribute to defence against infection.

3. Name three types of molecule (other than antibody) that contribute to defence against infection.

4. Name three natural immune components that contribute to acute inflammation.

5. Name three results of complement activation.

6. 'In general, the same natural immune mechanisms act against viruses and against bacteria.' Is this true?

7. 'Natural immune mechanisms are not exclusively used to combat infection.' Is this true?

8. Invertebrates survive very nicely with a natural immune system, but we vertebrates need adaptive immunity as well. Speculate on why this might be.

9. The immune system is there to interact with the world of infectious (parasitic) microorganisms. Where exactly is the interface between parasite and host?

Further reading

If you have the time and the interest, it is worth reading more widely about what has been covered in this section, starting with the following.

Bibel D J 1988 Milestones in immunology. Science-Tech 330 pp. A fascinating collection of classic papers, including Metchnikoff and Almroth Wright on phagocytosis, Bordet on complement, Dale on histamine, etc. with a well-informed modern appraisal. Wonderful reading.

Wilkinson P 1982 Chemotaxis and inflammation. Churchill Livingstone, Edinburgh, 249 pp. Everything you could possibly want to know about leucocyte movement.

Whaley K (ed) 1987 Complement in health and disease, MTP Press, 326 pp. A useful multi-expert summary of the role of complement in both infection and pathology.

Alberts B, Bray D, Lewis J, Raff M, Roberts K, Watson J D 1994 Molecular biology of the cell, 3rd edn. Garland Publishing, the Netherlands, 1294 pp. The Membrane Transport section of this classic book helps to put phagocytosis in the context of endocytosis in general.

Roitt I M 1994 Essential immunology, 8th edn. Blackwell Scientific, Oxford, 448 pp. The top British book on immunology, worth consulting for further detail on all aspects as you go through the course.

Janeway CA, Travers P 1994 Immunobiology. Current Biology Ltd, London, 643pp. A good new American book, well illustrated and referenced, emphasising basic principles.

Answers

1. Natural immune mechanisms act fast; show low specificity in both recognition and disposal; do not show memory. Adaptive immunity acts more slowly; shows very high specificity in recognition; shows memory (the secondary response); is restricted to vertebrates. (Note, however, that disposal is still largely via the mechanisms used by the natural immune system: complement, phagocytosis, etc.)

2. Macrophages secrete lysozyme and some complement components (anti-bacterial); they secrete interferon (anti-viral); they are phagocytic (mainly anti-bacterial); by secreting cytokines they induce the acute phase response.

3. The complement components; interferon; C-reactive protein. More indirectly: cytokines; histamine.

4. Anaphylotoxins (C3a, C5a); histamine; mast cells; PMN (via their enzymes).

5. Opsonization of particles for phagocytosis; puncture of cell membranes (lysis); promotion of inflammation.

6. In general, this statement is not true. The anti-viral mechanisms interferon and NK cells are less effective against non-viral organisms, while complement and phagocytes are more relevant to bacteria and fungi than to viruses. But it is not entirely untrue, since interferon *can* contribute to defence against bacteria, fungi and protozoa, while viruses *can* sometimes be disposed of by phagocytosis or complement-mediated lysis.

7. Yes. Phagocytes take up many non-microbial objects, e.g. carbon particles in the airways. The acute phase and inflammatory responses are involved in repair and healing of injury, even when the wound is completely sterile. IFN and NK cells *may* have a role in controlling cancer. Handling infection is just one of the functions of the natural immune system, but a very important one.

8. This is a difficult one. You can think of features of some vertebrates that might make infection a larger problem than for some invertebrates (greater size; longer lifespan; land habitat; higher body temperature) but few that distinguish all vertebrates from all invertebrates. The evolution of adaptive immunity involved some very complex gene duplications and rearrangements to make the receptors characteristic of lymphocytes and it may be sheer coincidence that this began around the time (about 550 million years ago) that the first vertebrates emerged. But higher vertebrates do undoubtedly need lymphocytes for good health, as is shown by the very delicate state of mice or humans born without them, whereas invertebrates seem to manage without. Note, however, that cells with *some* of the properties of lymphocytes can be found in invertebrates.

9. Parasite and host interact at the level of the recognition molecules of the immune system. These include the receptors on phagocytic and NK cells (mainly carbohydrate), the alternative complement pathway components and the antigen receptors on lymphocytes. The last are by far the most discriminatory (specific) as well as being the best understood, and will be described in the next section.

The Lymphocyte and Lymphoid Tissue

As mentioned earlier, a new kind of immune cell emerged during evolution — the **lymphocyte** — which was different from the cells of the natural immune system in that it had the property of *specificity* for particular microbial antigens and the development of *memory*. It has been estimated that we have around 10^{12} lymphocytes. If lumped together this would be equivalent to about the size of a football!

Morphology and organization of lymphocytes

Lymphocytes are mononuclear cells and in their resting state have a thin rim of cytoplasm (Fig. 1*a*) generally containing very few cytoplasmic organelles, as seen by electron microscopy (Fig. 1*b*). They are found in encapsulated lymphoid organs, in aggregates of lymphoid tissues and in the circulation. The **lymphoid organs/tissues** contain other cell populations (**accessory cells**) which are required for their function. The major lymphoid organs/tissues (shown in Fig. 2) are generally classified into **primary** (central) or **secondary** (peripheral).

Primary lymphoid organs

Like all blood cells, lymphocytes are produced by the process of differentiation from a common haemopoietic stem cell (HSC). This cell gives rise to the lymphoid stem cell (LSC), which is now committed to differentiate into lymphocytes rather than granulocytes, red cells, etc. (Fig. 3).

The primary organs provide the micro-environments for the two major lymphocyte types or subsets (T and B) to develop from stem cells immigrating from the blood stream. T lymphocytes develop in the **thymus**, a bilobed organ situated in the thorax overlying the major blood vessels. Each thymic lobule contains an outer **cortex** and an inner **medulla** (see your histology textbook for more details). Differentiation and selection of the newly produced T cells occurs through interactions with specialized endothelial cells and macrophages and follows a cortico-medullary direction, the more mature cells being found in the medulla. The **bone marrow** is the site of development of the **B lymphocytes**. In both the thymus and the bone marrow, many lymphocytes die (commit suicide!), only a small number of selected cells being allowed to leave via the blood stream to seed the secondary lymphoid tissues (p. 21).

Secondary lymphoid organs and tissues

Lymphocytes carry out their function in the secondary lymphoid organs and tissues. The **spleen** is composed of red pulp and white pulp (Fig. 4). The white pulp is also referred to as the peri-arteriolar lymphoid sheath (**PALS**) since the lymphocytes in it usually surround an arteriolar branch of the splenic artery. The outer layer of the PALS — the marginal zone — contains many macrophages and is the port of entry of lymphocytes from the circulation. Many phagocytic macrophages are present in the red pulp which is also the main site for **plasma cell** development. The spleen is the main lymphoid organ for protection against blood-borne antigens mainly via the action of macrophages in the red pulp.

Lymph nodes (Fig. 5) are found throughout the body. They vary from 1 to 15 mm in size and each is composed of an outer cortex (B cell area) and inner medulla (containing T, B cells and plasma cells). The deep cortex or paracortical region contains mainly T cells (T cell area). Specialized antigen-presenting cells (APC) which interact with either B or T cells are found in the cortex and paracortical regions, respectively. The siting of the lymph nodes at junctions of the lymphatic vessels allows them to 'filter out' and deal with micro-organisms washed up the lymphatics from the **interstitial tissues**.

In addition to being the primary site of B cell production, the bone marrow in man is also a secondary lymphoid organ containing many plasma cells (p. 17).

Over half of the total lymphoid cells of the body are found in the lamina propria and submucosal sites of the gastrointestinal, respiratory and genito-urinary tracts, i.e. lining the surfaces of externally opening organs. These are referred to collectively as the mucosa-associated lymphoid tissue (**MALT**). In the intestine, some lymphoid aggregations may be very large and are called **Peyer's patches**. The tonsils in man also consist mainly of lymphocytes.

Secondary follicles with **germinal centres** are a common feature of secondary lymphoid organs/tissues and are the site of memory B cell responses (p. 29).

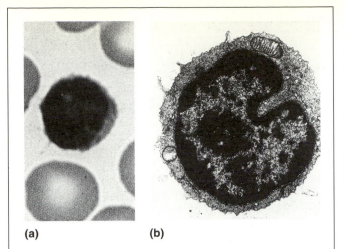

Fig. 1 The lymphocyte. A 'resting' blood lymphocyte **(a)** stained with Giemsa. Note the small amount of cytoplasm and organelles as shown in **(b)**, the electron micrograph.

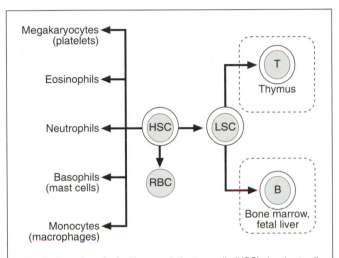

Fig. 3 Lymphopoiesis. Haemopoietic stem cells (HSC) give rise to all the different cells of the blood (haemopoiesis). Some of these HSC become lymphoid stem cells (LSC) which differentiate into T and B lymphocytes in the thymus and bone marrow respectively (the process of lymphopoiesis).

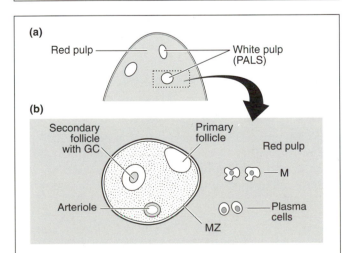

Fig. 4 The spleen. (a) The spleen is composed of red and white pulp. The white pulp (lymphoid tissue) is organized around blood vessels. This periarteriolar lymphoid sheath (PALS) **(b)** consists of lymphocyte aggregate (primary follicles) and secondary follicles containing dividing B lymphocytes (germinal centres: GC). The PALS is separated from the red pulp by a marginal zone (MZ). The red pulp contains macrophages (M) and plasma cells (not drawn to scale).

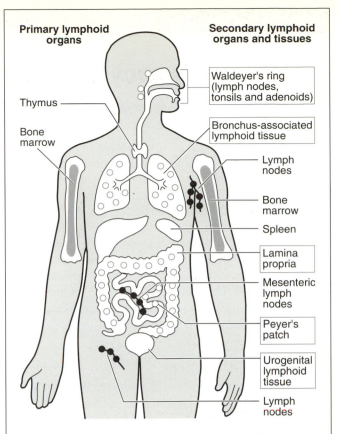

Fig. 2 The major lymphoid organs and tissues. The mucosa-associated lymphoid tissue is shown in boxes. We have a large amount of MALT since the mucosal surface area is about 400 times the external surface area of the body and is without the outer protective epidermal layer of the skin.

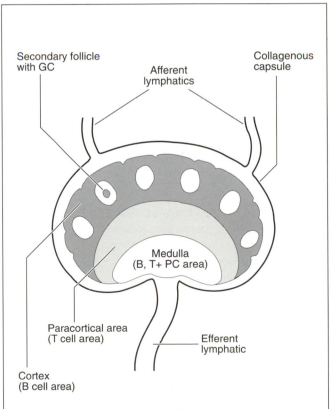

Fig. 5 A lymph node. Each lymph node is surrounded by a collagenous capsule. T cells are found mainly in the deep cortex or paracortical area. Lymph enters via the afferent lymphatics, is filtered as it passes through the node and emerges through the efferent lymphatic to eventually join the lymph in the thoracic duct.

B and T Lymphocytes

Even though B and T lymphocytes have different jobs to do in the adaptive immune response, they have a number of properties in common:

- Unlike all other blood cells, they *recirculate* around the body from blood to tissues and back again into the circulation. In lymph nodes, lymphocytes leave the circulation by attaching through 'homing' receptors to **high endothelial cells** (**HEC**) of the **post capillary venules** (**PCV**) and passing between them. Lymphocyte recirculation allows them to home to the different sites in the body where they can encounter antigen (Fig. 1).
- Each lymphocyte has individual receptors in its plasma membrane to enable it to recognize a particular antigen. This is what confers *specificity* on the lymphocyte.
- They undergo **clonal proliferation** when they are 'activated' by their specific receptor making contact with its specific antigen (p. 27).
- They show the property of **memory**, giving rise to a faster and bigger immune response on re-challenge with the same antigen.

However, B and T lymphocytes also differ in many respects.

B lymphocytes

Although T and B lymphocytes look alike under normal histological stains, they can be distinguished from one another by virtue of the fact that they have different functional molecules associated with them. For example, B lymphocytes but *not* T lymphocytes have **immunoglobulins** (antibodies) on their surface which act as antigen receptors (see p. 19). These can be detected using specific antibodies to human immunoglobulin labelled with fluorescent dyes which 'light up' the surface of the B cells (but not T cells) when the lymphocytes with bound antibodies are exposed to ultraviolet light (UV). They can be quantitated under the UV microscope (Fig. 2) or by using a laser-based **flow cytometer** (see p. 92). Other surface molecules unique to B lymphocytes are detectable by the appropriate fluorescent antibodies, e.g. CD19, CD20 (see Appendix 3 for table of CD markers).

When mature B lymphocytes are stimulated through their antigen receptors they develop into antibody secreting **plasma cells** (antibody 'factories', Fig. 3). These cells are rich in organelles associated with protein synthesis, i.e. rough endoplasmic reticulum and mitochondria. Plasma cells, despite their name, are normally found in the lymphoid tissues and only at very low levels in the circulation. Alternatively, the stimulated B cells may develop into memory B lymphocytes. B lymphocytes also act as antigen-presenting cells (APC) to T lymphocytes (p. 31).

T lymphocytes: two functional subpopulations

Two distinct T lymphocyte subpopulations are produced in the thymus. Correspondingly, when they recognize their antigen, they respond by clonal proliferation and carry out one of two functions:

- They help/amplify the immune response (**helper T cells, T_H cells, CD4 cells**), mainly by cytokine production (see p. 33) or
- They kill cells bearing the antigen (**cytotoxic T cells, T_C, CD8 cells**; see p. 35).

During development, thymocytes co-express CD4 and CD8 molecules (double positives, Fig. 4) but the mature cells emerge from the thymus as either CD4 or CD8 (single positives) and retain these markers when they migrate into the secondary lymphoid tissues and respond to antigens. The CD4 and CD8 molecules guide the T cell to the appropriate target by interacting with MHC class II and class I molecules, respectively.

Other surface molecules on T lymphocytes

CD3 is present on the surface of all T lymphocytes and is associated with the T cell antigen receptor (p. 19). **CD2** molecules are expressed by T cells (but also by natural killer cells). The **CD5** molecule is also expressed by the majority of T cells and, like CD2 and CD3, is an accessory molecule for activation of T cells (p. 28).

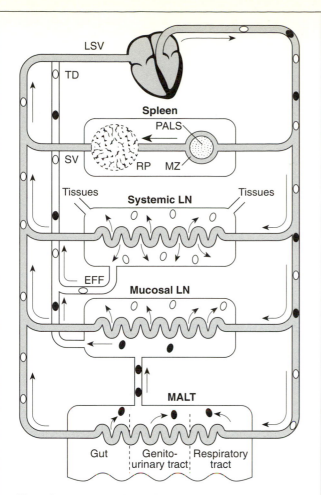

Fig. 1 Lymphocyte traffic and recirculation. Lymphocytes (0) enter the PALS via the marginal zone (MZ) and leave through the splenic vein (SV) in the red pulp (RP). Lymphocytes enter the lymph node from the tissues but mainly through the post capillary venules located in the cortical-paracortical junction. They leave the node via the efferent lymphatics (EFF) and reach the large thoracic duct (TD) which empties its contents back into the circulation at the left subclavian vein (LSV). The mucosal lymphocyte recirculatory system is unique in that lymphocytes stimulated, for example, in the gut mucosal surfaces pass into the draining lymph nodes and hence via the EFF and TD back into the circulation. (●) These lymphocytes 'home' back to all three mucosal areas thus protecting all mucosal surfaces from reinfection.

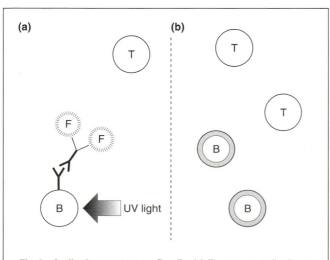

Fig. 2 Antibody receptors on B cells. (a) Fluorescent antibodies to human immunoglobulin (F) bind to B cells but not T cells. On exposure to ultraviolet light, the fluorescein emits green light which can be seen under the fluorescence microscope (b) and the B cells identified.

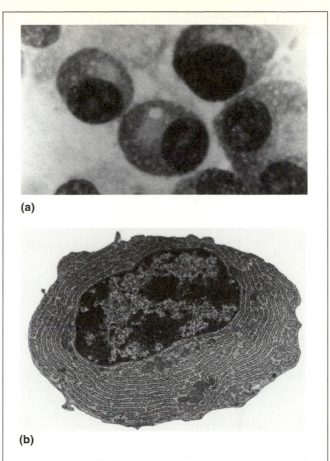

Fig. 3 Plasma cells. Plasma cells have more cytoplasm than their B lymphocyte precursors (a). (b) At the ultrastructural level, one can see mitochondria and extensive rough endoplasmic reticulum, the machinery required for high rates of antibody synthesis.

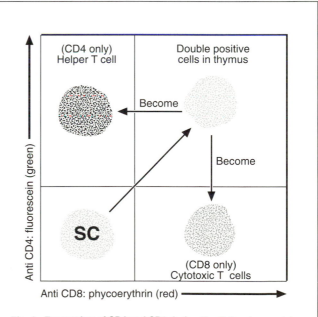

Fig. 4 Expression of CD4 and CD8 during T cell development. In the thymus, the immigrant stem cell (SC) expresses neither CD4 nor CD8. During early differentiation, the T cells express both CD4 and CD8 on their surface (often called double positive cells). These then lose either CD4 to become CD8 cytotoxic T cells or CD8 to become CD4 helper T cells. The cells leave the thymus to function in the secondary lymphoid organs and tissues. Here the lymphocytes are stained simultaneously with antibodies to CD4 (fluorescein, green) and CD8 (phycoerythrin, red). The stained cells were analysed by flow cytometry (p. 91). Each dot represents a single cell.

Recognition Molecules

The function of the immune system is to recognize and dispose of invading microbes. In the adaptive immune system, each lymphocyte has a unique recognition structure which allows it to 'see' antigen. These **receptors** are present in high numbers on the surface of lymphocytes (around 10^5 per cell) and are glycoproteins, as are many other receptors such as those recognising hormones (see your biochemistry textbook). The *three* main specific recognition structures of the adaptive immune system are:

- antibody
- **T cell receptor (TCR)**
- class I and II **major histocompatibility complex (MHC)** molecules.

All three of these groups of protein share a common origin in evolution: they are members of the **immunoglobulin super-family**. Folding of the molecule (secondary structure) results in the formation of a groove able to bind a **ligand**. As in hormone–receptor interactions, binding to the ligand is *non-covalent* and reversible, obeying the laws of mass action. It involves every known non-covalent bond: van der Waal's bonds (induced dipoles), hydrophobic interactions and charge interactions.

B cell antigen receptors

The antigen receptors of B lymphocytes are glycoproteins called antibodies (immunoglobulin; Ig). They are composed of two heavy and two light chains, each with a *variable* and a *constant* region. Two other kinds of molecule, Igα and Igβ, are associated with the antibody molecule, and together they make up the **B cell receptor complex** (Fig. 1). Most B lymphocytes express surface Ig of two classes: IgM and IgD. Note that it is the monomeric and not pentameric form of IgM antibody which is the antigen receptor on the B cell surface (see p. 23).

T cell antigen receptors

Most T lymphocytes have antigen receptor molecules composed of two different polypeptide chains (α and β) held together by disulphide bonds. A minor population of T lymphocytes uses two other polypeptide chains: γ and δ. As with antibody, these polypeptide chains have variable (V) and constant regions (C). A group of five separate polypeptides (**CD3**) are associated with the heterodimer and together this is called the **TCR complex** (Fig. 2).

Receptor diversity: gene rearrangement

The outer domains of each of the antibody light (L) and heavy (H) chains, and TCR α and β chains, are variable in their amino acid sequence. The antibody variable regions are the products of 2L and 3H minigenes (Fig. 3). During early B cell development, the several hundred germ-line minigenes are randomly rearranged on the chromosomes and, together with the addition of nucleotides and errors in joining, result in the production of polypeptides with extremely variable amino acid sequences. The random association of H and L chains further increases the repertoire diversity. The constant region domains are coded for by one gene which determines the antibody class. A similar kind of rearrangement of minigenes (two α and three β) occurs for the TCR. This type of rearrangement is unique to lymphocytes, and results in a single polypeptide coded by several genes instead of the normal 'one gene one polypeptide' rule.

MHC molecules

The T cell receptor, unlike antibody on B cells, only recognizes antigen when it is associated with specific 'receptor molecules' (MHC molecules, Fig. 4) on the surface of cells. The two major types of MHC molecules are **class I** (found on *all nucleated cells* of the body) and **class II** found on a limited number of specialized **antigen-presenting cells**. Protein antigens have to be broken up into smaller pieces (processed) by proteases within the cell and then presented as small peptides in the groove of MHC molecules. In the case of endogenous antigens such as viral proteins the processed peptides become associated with MHC class I molecules; those antigens taken in by the process of endocytosis (e.g. by macrophages or B cells) associate with MHC class II molecules. Note: MHC stands for major histocompatibility complex, a name given when the importance of the MHC in **graft rejection** was realized (see p. 51).

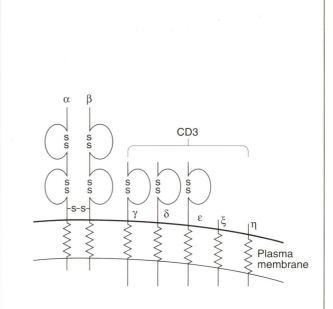

Fig. 1 The B cell receptor complex. IgM is the initial antigen receptor. IgD is found in addition to IgM on most mature B cells. The accessory molecules Igα and Igβ form heterodimers which are non-covalently associated with IgM in the membrane. These molecules are involved in activation of the B cell.

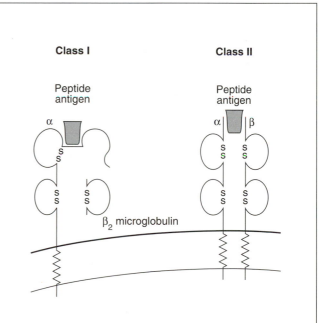

Fig. 2 The T cell receptor complex. Two disulphide-linked polypeptide chains make up this heterodimer (two 'unlike' chains). Two different polypeptide chains γ and δ form the TCR in a minority of T cells. The TCR is associated with five different chains (CD3). These are involved in T cell activation.

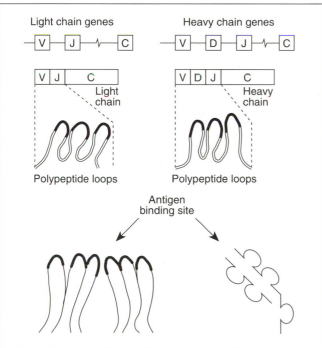

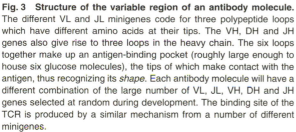

Fig. 3 Structure of the variable region of an antibody molecule. The different VL and JL minigenes code for three polypeptide loops which have different amino acids at their tips. The VH, DH and JH genes also give rise to three loops in the heavy chain. The six loops together make up an antigen-binding pocket (roughly large enough to house six glucose molecules), the tips of which make contact with the antigen, thus recognizing its *shape*. Each antibody molecule will have a different combination of the large number of VL, JL, VH, DH and JH genes selected at random during development. The binding site of the TCR is produced by a similar mechanism from a number of different minigenes.

Fig. 4 MHC molecules. The two outer domains of the α chain of the MHC class I molecule form a groove into which the antigenic peptide fits. This chain is associated non-covalently with a small polypeptide, β2 microglobulin, which is essential for surface expression of the α chain. The α (33 kDa) and β (28 kDa) chains of the MHC class II molecule are held together by non-covalent bonds. The outer domains of each chain form a groove which binds the antigenic peptide. Both class I and class II grooves consist of 2 α-helices with a floor of β-pleated sheets.

Self Versus Non-self Discrimination

The question at the heart of immunology

As already emphasized, the immune system has evolved to recognize and dispose of foreign microbes. But how does the immune system know what is foreign? In other words, how does it distinguish its own cells and tissues (*self*) from the microbial invaders (*non-self*)? In fact there are several answers to this question.

The natural immune system

As discussed later, the ultimate disposal mechanism for microbes is the phagocyte. The failure to phagocytose our own normal cells is due to the fact that they are coated with certain surface sugars which are not recognized by the cells of the phagocytic system. In some cases, e.g. red cells, gradual 'damage' to these carbohydrate surfaces eventually allows the ageing cell to be recognized and phagocytosed. Microbes do not have these particular sugars but do have others which macrophages normally recognize. A rather similar mechanism operates within the complement system.

The adaptive immune system

Each T and B lymphocyte carries surface receptors which are specific for a given antigen by means of which a huge range of foreign antigens are recognized. These receptors could potentially also recognize self-antigens since microbes are made up of many of the carbohydrates, proteins and lipids which constitute our own tissues (remember, we all use the same 20 amino acids!). There is no way in which the information to make these 'self-reactive' receptors could be obliterated from our DNA. Nevertheless, in most cases, lymphocytes are fortunately unable to respond to self-antigens and we are said to be unresponsive, or *tolerant* of our own antigens.

There are two levels at which this tolerance can occur: **central** and **peripheral**.

Central tolerance

Central tolerance is the elimination of self-reactive cells during lymphocyte development. Most of our knowledge about central tolerance has come from the study of T cell development, so this will be described here. As we have previously indicated and will be describing in detail later (p. 31), the T cell receptor only recognizes processed antigens bound to cell surface MHC molecules. Each receptor specificity is generated randomly from a pool of germ-line genes as the lymphoid stem cells differentiate. There is then a process which selects, for subsequent use, only those cells weakly recognizing MHC molecules (Fig. 1, **positive selection**). Since the process of receptor generation is random, receptor specificities are inevitably produced which will bind to self-antigenic determinants associated with MHC molecules. But as new lymphocytes appear bearing receptors with a sufficiently high affinity to attach to self-peptide–MHC complexes, they are 'activated', not into clonal proliferation (as described on p. 27) but to commit suicide. This process is referred to as **negative selection**, and the cells die through **apoptosis**, which is also known as 'programmed cell death' and is the normal way body cells die (e.g. in the brain, liver, etc.). It is due to activation of degradative enzymes which cut the DNA into defined lengths, the hallmark of this mechanism of cell death. A similar process of negative selection is thought to occur during the development of B cells.

Peripheral tolerance

Peripheral tolerance is the unresponsiveness of self-reactive cells outside the primary lymphoid organs. Some T cells with low affinity, or low numbers of receptors, for self-antigens escape negative selection. Moreover, not all self-antigens are present in, or pass through, the primary lymphoid organs and, therefore, lymphocytes with the corresponding specificity escape suicide. These lymphocytes are normally kept in an unresponsive state in two main ways, known as **clonal anergy** and **ignorance** (see Fig. 2 for more details).

Breakdown in tolerance to self-antigens by either T or B cells leads to **autoimmunity** and sometimes autoimmune disease, as described on page 47.

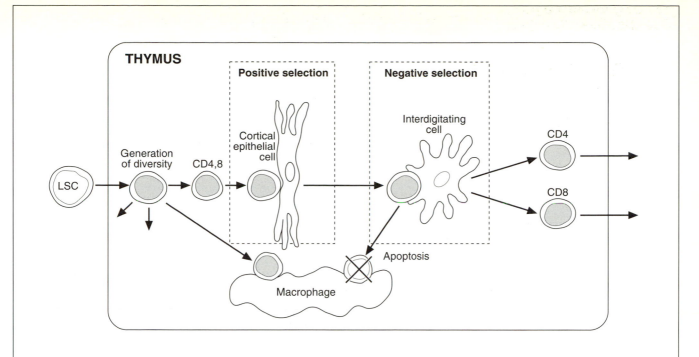

Fig. 1 Mechanisms of central tolerance. Lymphoid stem cells enter the thymus and begin their development into T cells. The first stage is the generation of the different receptors for antigen by each cell (generation of diversity). Some of these cells fail to express functional receptors and die, to be removed by macrophages. Cells bearing receptors with low affinity for self-MHC molecules alone interact with cortical epithelial cells and are *positively* selected to survive. These cells express low levels of both CD4 and CD8. In the second selection stage, cells bearing receptors with high affinity for self-peptide–MHC complexes, displayed on interdigitating cells, are *negatively* selected by being made to commit suicide; these dying cells are removed by macrophages. The remaining cells lose either CD4 or CD8 and leave the thymus to function in the periphery as mature T cells.

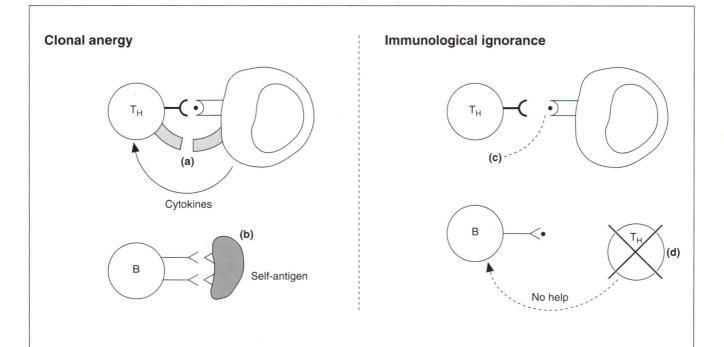

Fig. 2 Mechanisms of peripheral tolerance. There are several ways in which self-reactive lymphocytes in the periphery can be kept unresponsive. (1) **Clonal anergy**: (a) T cells fail to respond to autoantigens because they do not receive appropriate co-stimulatory signals mediated by accessory molecules (p. 27); (b) B cells, at the early stage when they express low levels of IgM and high levels of IgD (p. 19), respond to high levels of self-antigen by becoming unresponsive. (2) **Immunological ignorance**: (c) Self-reactive T cells are not activated by self-antigens present in small amounts; these include 'sequestered' antigens such as lens and sperm proteins. Alternatively, there might be too little self-peptide on MHC molecules for T cells with low numbers of receptors to respond — a 'threshold' effect. (d) At the B cell level, it is much more difficult to show ignorance to self-antigens; these probably fail to induce high-affinity autoantibodies mainly through lack of help from self-reactive T cells. Thus T cell tolerance is the mainstay of self-unresponsiveness.

Antibody

As you will remember from the discussion of recognition molecules (p. 19), antibodies are glycosylated proteins with a basic composition of two heavy and two light polypeptide chains. A three-dimensional model of an antibody molecule is illustrated in Figure 1 (see your biochemistry notes on protein structure). The N-terminal outer domains of each chain form the **antigen-binding site** and since there are two of these for each antibody 'monomer' this region is called the F(ab)$_2$ region. At the other end, the Fc region is formed from the two identical heavy chains and determines the 'biological activity' of the antibody. For this purpose, there are *five* classes of antibodies which are based on the isotypes of the heavy chain used. There are also two light chain isotypes, κ and λ. Only one light chain and one heavy chain isotype can be used by each antibody molecule.

The combination of antibody and antigen is known as an **immune complex**. You will come across this term again, in relation to both beneficial and harmful immunity.

Antibody class and function

Each antibody class is structurally adapted for a particular biological activity and functions best at a different site in the body. This is why there are several genes for the H chain of the constant region.

IgM is a large protein (macroglobulin) made up of five identical monomeric subunits held together by a small protein (J chain, Fig. 2a) and largely confined to the circulation. It is also present in the monomeric form on the surface of most B lymphocytes (see p. 19). The secreted form is predominant in early immune responses to most antigens and provides an effective first line defence against bacteraemia (Fig. 2b). Although each subunit has a low **affinity** for antigen, its pentameric structure gives the whole molecule a relatively high **avidity**. The affinity is a measure of the strength of binding of a single binding unit to an antigenic shape or '**epitope**', whereas the avidity is the strength of binding of the entire antibody molecule with its multiple binding sites to several identical epitopes of an antigen. The multiple binding sites of IgM allow it to attach to several identical epitopes on different particulate antigens simultaneously, leading to agglutination. Blood group antibodies are mainly of this class.

IgD is present predominantly as a monomer, together with IgM, on the surface of most B lymphocytes. Its function is at present unclear but it probably acts as an antigen receptor for the control of lymphocyte activation and suppression. It is thought to be absent from memory cells.

IgG is the predominant immunoglobulin in the blood stream and tissue fluids, where it combats microorganisms and their toxins. There are four subclasses of IgG, all monomeric. IgG antibodies generally have a higher affinity for antigens than IgM. As well as being able to pass from blood to tissues, IgG is the only class of antibody to cross the placenta and this provides the newborn child with useful protection against infections to which the mother is immune (Fig. 3).

IgA exists in both monomeric and dimeric forms (two monomers held together by a J chain, Fig. 4a). It is monomeric in the circulation. In its polymeric form it provides the primary defence against 'local' infections owing to its abundance in saliva, tears, bronchial secretions, nasal mucosa, prostatic fluid, vaginal secretions and mucous secretions of the small intestine. Secretory IgA is transported across epithelial surfaces and released with a secretory piece into the exterior lumen (gut, genito-urinary tract, etc., Fig. 4b). The level of IgA in secretions increases rapidly after birth to provide similar protection at the mucosal surface to that afforded by IgG in the circulation. IgA antibodies in breast milk colostrum may also protect the baby during early life. There are two subclasses of IgA.

IgE is present as a monomer at very low levels in the circulation but provides protection for external body surfaces, especially mucosal surfaces, by recruiting anti-microbial cells and agents. Mast cells have high affinity receptors for the Fc region of IgE. The IgE-mediated degranulation of the mast cell, on exposure to its antigen, enhances the acute inflammatory response by recruiting a variety of cells into the site of infection. Levels of this antibody, normally very low, are increased during worm infections and this class of antibody probably evolved for protection against such intruders. On the negative side, IgE is responsible for the symptoms of atopic allergy (p. 45).

The properties of the different classes and subclasses of antibodies are summarized in Figure 5.

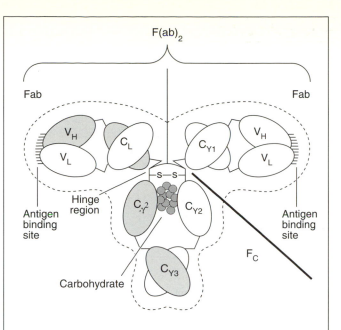

Fig. 1 **Schematic diagram of IgG** (from crystallographic studies). This shows the interactions of the heavy and light chain domains. Note the antigen-binding sites and the hinge region which gives the molecule flexibility (see Fig. 2b). Fab and Fc regions are indicated.

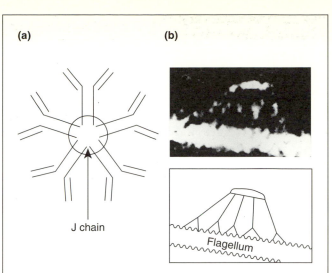

Fig. 2 **IgM molecule.** The five subunits of IgM are held together by a J chain (**a**). The electron micrograph shows this large molecule attached in 'spider' form to its antigen, a bacterial flagellum (**b**).

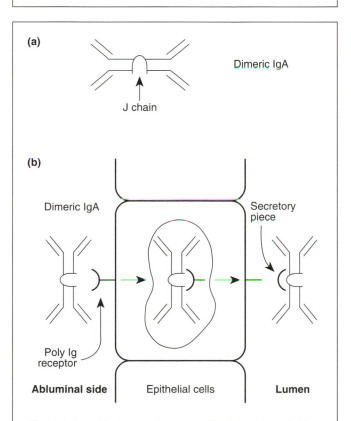

Fig. 4 **IgA and its transport across epithelial surfaces. (a)** Two (and sometimes more) IgA molecules are held together by a J chain. These attach to poly Ig receptors on the abluminal epithelial surface (**b**), are transported via endosomes and are released together with a piece of the receptor (secretory piece) into the lumen.

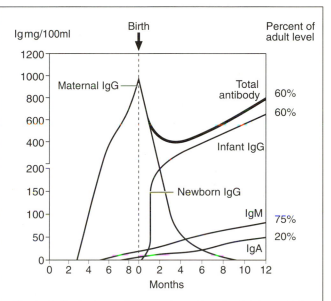

Fig. 3 **Antibody classes in the newborn.** Note the high level of IgG (maternal) at birth.

Immuno-globulin	Mol. wt. (kDa)	Heavy chain	Serum* conc. mg/ml⁻¹	Complement fixation	Placental transfer	Binding to Mθ/ PMNs
IgM	900	μ	1.5	++	–	–
IgD	184	δ	0.03	–	–	–
IgG1	146	γ^1	9	++	+	++
IgG2	146	γ^2	3	+	+/–	+
IgG3	170	γ^3	1	++	+	++
IgG4	146	γ^4	0.5	+/–	+	+/–
IgA1	160	α^1	3	?	–	±
IgA2	160	α^2	0.5	?	–	±
IgE	188	ε	50 (ng/ml)	–	–	+**

Fig. 5 **Summary of the properties of the antibody classes and sub-classes.** *Mean conc; **Mast cells. Note that antibodies have quite a short half-life in the circulation: about 21 days for IgG, 10 days for IgM and only 6 days for IgA.

Tutorial 2

You should now be familiar with the special features of the lymphocyte, especially those that make it the cornerstone of the adaptive immune system. You should also know something about the recognition molecules of adaptive immunity, particularly antibody. The following questions will test your knowledge. Check your answers with the ones on the opposite page.

Questions

1. What properties distinguish lymphocytes from other cells involved in immunity?

2. What functional features distinguish B from T lymphocytes?

3. How can B and T lymphocytes be distinguished in the laboratory?

4. Distinguish between primary and secondary lymphoid organs.

5. What do antibodies, T cell receptors and MHC molecules have in common?

6. Why do we have so many classes of antibody?

7. What do you understand by the term immune complex?

8. Why is it that we do not normally make immune responses against our own molecules?

9. Why do you think there are two sets (classes) of MHC molecules?

Further reading

All the comprehensive immunology textbooks cover adaptive immunity very thoroughly. Essential immunology has already been mentioned; here are some other good books, varying mainly in size and detail, but each, of course, possessing its own flavour.

Male D 1991 Immunology, 2nd edn. Gower Medical, London, 128 pp. A useful dictionary-style booklet which actually (for once!) does fit into the pocket.

Playfair J H L 1992 Immunology at a glance, 5th edn. Blackwell Scientific, Oxford. Another short book with 43 'spreads', aimed at the busy student, scientist, layman, etc.

Kuby J 1994 Immunology, 2nd edn. W H Freeman, Oxford, 660 pp. A fine new American book, covering the whole field with clear Scientific American style diagrams and an emphasis on study questions (with answers).

Hood L E, Weissman I L, Wood W B, Wilson J H, 1984 Immunology, 2nd edn. Benjamin/Cummings. Not quite up-to-date now, but an excellent all-round text.

Klein J 1990 Immunology. Blackwell Scientific, Oxford, 508 pp. Another good overview of the subject, by one of the pioneers of immunogenetics.

Roitt I M, Brostoff J, Male D 1993 Immunology, 3nd edn. Gower Medical, London. A multi-author book with hundreds of vivid pictures, also available as a slide atlas.

The reader interested in being really up-to-date (remember, most text books are about 2 years old when they appear), should keep an eye on the following journals:

Immunology Today; Immunology; Clinical and Experimental Immunology; Journal of Immunology; Journal of Experimental Medicine; Nature; Lancet; European Journal of Immunology; Proceedings of the National Academy of Sciences, USA; Science; Cell.

Answers

1. They carry surface receptors with very high specificity for antigens, coded for by minigenes which have to be rearranged to produce a functional molecule. When activated, they proliferate rapidly into clones. They can develop into memory cells and thus mediate secondary responses. They recirculate through both blood and tissues. No other cell displays these properties. In addition, as compared to macrophages and PMN, they are not phagocytic.

2. The function of B lymphocytes is to monitor the extracellular compartments of the body, to recognize foreign antigens, and to make antibody against them. This requires recognition of their three-dimensional shape. The function of T cells is to monitor the intracellular compartments of the body, to recognize small peptides derived from microbes contained therein, and to act accordingly: either by killing the cell (if it contains a virus), to help its own killing processes (e.g. if it is a macrophage) or to help it proliferate and make antibody (if it is a B cell).

3. By demonstrating the presence of their characteristic surface molecules (or 'markers'). For B cells, surface immunoglobulin is easiest to show, by reacting the cell with fluorescein-labelled anti-human Ig antibody and examining it under UV light. Other B cell-specific markers include CD 19 and 20. For T cells the most useful marker is CD3, with CD4 and CD8 for the two subpopulations.

4. Primary lymphoid organs are where the precursors differentiate into mature cells: for T cells the thymus and for B cells the bone marrow (and liver in the fetus). Secondary lymphoid organs are where the mature cells reside and function: for both T and B cells these include the spleen, lymph nodes, Peyer's patches, tonsils, etc.

5. They share a characteristic 'domain' structure and demonstrate considerable homologies in both DNA and amino acid sequences. Therefore, they are considered to have evolved from a common precursor and are classified together in the 'Ig superfamily', which also includes important lymphocyte surface molecules such as CD3, CD4, CD8, some cytokine receptors and receptors for IgG, all of which are involved in cell–cell interactions.

6. Each antibody class has some particular protective value, because not all microorganisms can be dealt with in the same way. For example, IgM, being a large molecule (around 900 kDa), is mainly restricted to the circulation and protects against blood-borne microbes; IgA, through its secretory property and resistance to proteolysis, can function at mucosal surfaces; IgG permeates the tissues, protects the fetus and newborn and is the antibody which shows the greatest degree of affinity maturation.

7. An immune complex is simply what is formed when antibody binds to antigen. Remember this is not a covalent bond, but involves only physical forces. While immune complex formation is an essential part of antigen disposal, immune complexes can also, in certain circumstances, give rise to tissue damage (p. 45).

8. We are said to be 'tolerant' of our own molecules. First, this tolerance is achieved by elimination of B and T lymphocytes with specific receptors for self-antigens during development in the primary lymphoid organs (also referred to as 'negative selection'). Second, self-reactive lymphocytes which do not come into contact with their antigen in early development are maintained in a state of anergy by a number of different mechanisms (p. 21). Breakdown of this anergic state may give rise to autoimmunity and autoimmune disease, usually in later life (p. 47).

9. The two classes of MHC molecule correspond to the two types of T cell. Class I, by interacting with the CD8 molecule, informs cytotoxic T cells of the presence of a cell which needs to be killed. Class II, by interacting with CD4, informs helper T cells of a cell that could benefit from help. Because any cell can harbour a virus, class I is on all cells (except red cells). Because only certain cells can benefit from help, class II is restricted to these cells (antigen-presenting cells, macrophages, B cells, some activated T cells).

Lymphocyte Activation and Clonal Selection

Both T and B lymphocytes need to be stimulated into action (activated) in order to carry out their function. Recognition of antigen by a lymphocyte through the TCR or antibody receptor on B cells is the first stage of this process and results in **signal transduction** leading to movement of the lymphocyte from the resting G0 stage to G1 of the cell cycle. Subsequent to this, co-stimulatory signals are required to drive the T or B cell into cell division and differentiation.

B lymphocyte activation

The kind of antigen determines how B lymphocytes are activated.

- **Thymus-independent antigens.** You will remember that B cell receptors (antibodies) recognize conformational structure or shape of antigenic epitopes. Large molecules with repetitive antigenic determinants (epitopes), e.g. some bacterial cell surface polysaccharides, cross-link the receptors and, thus, activate the B cells (Fig. 1). This is thought to occur in the marginal zones of the splenic PALS (p. 15). In addition, endotoxins from Gram-negative bacteria can bind directly to B cells through lipid A and this results in activation of all B cells, independent of their individual specificities.

- **Thymus-dependent antigens.** Antigens such as proteins, with single antigenic determinants, cannot directly activate B cells. They require help from T cells. The B cells endocytose the antigen through their antibody receptors, degrade it and present it to T cells bound with surface MHC class II molecules (p. 31). This interaction with the T cell results in B cell activation (Fig. 1). A number of **accessory molecules** on the surfaces of both the T cells and B cells are important for the activation process of both types of cells (Fig. 2).

T cell activation

CD4+ T cells are activated when their receptors bind degraded antigens (peptides) in association with MHC class II as presented on B cells (see above) or on other antigen-presenting cells including some dendritic cells and macrophages. CD8+ cytotoxic T cells are activated in a similar way when their receptors bind to peptides associated with class I MHC molecules.

Biochemical events involved in initial activation

You will have read in your cell biology textbook that a number of intracellular messengers are involved in carrying the signal generated through cell surface receptors to the nucleus. The same applies to lymphocytes and a summary of these pathways and 'second messengers' is shown in Figure 3. Co-stimulatory signals are required to drive the B and T cells into cell cycle and complete the differentiation process. T cells produce growth factors (cytokines, p. 33) which the B cells require to increase in number and develop into memory and antibody-secreting plasma cells (p. 29). T cells also require additional cytokine signals from themselves (autocrine, e.g. IL-2) and from antigen-presenting cells (e.g. IL-1) in order to proliferate.

Clonal selection

Even the smallest microbe will have several different foreign antigenic epitopes and all those lymphocytes with corresponding receptors will be activated. This will still amount to only a fraction of the whole lymphocyte population: perhaps 1/10 000 – 1/100 000 of the total repertoire of T and B cells (Fig. 4). The activated cells, stimulated by cytokines, increase in number. This results in selection of clones of B and T cells, each of which has identical surface receptors for antigen. Some members of the clone become memory cells and, in the case of B cells, some differentiate into antibody-secreting plasma cells. This process takes place in the **germinal centres** of the secondary follicles (p. 29). Helper and cytotoxic T cells recognizing their specific antigenic determinants bound to MHC molecules are clonally selected in a similar fashion. Memory T cells are also produced in this process.

Since many different clones are activated in response to the antigens carried by each microbe, a typical B or T response is **polyclonal**. Monoclonal reponses are extremely rare, but **monoclonal antibodies** can be made by a special technique.

T cell independent activation | **T cell dependent activation**

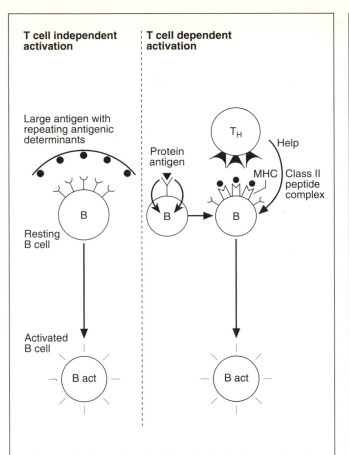

Fig. 1 Activation of B cells (B_{act}) via the T-independent and T-dependent pathways. For more details of the T – B cell interactions, see Figure 2.

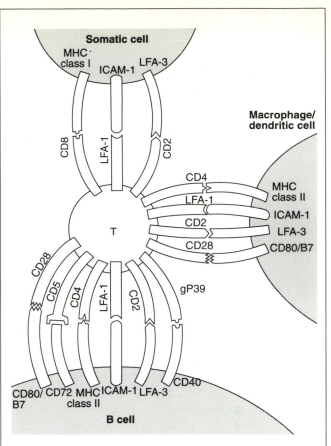

Fig. 2 Numerous accessory molecules are involved in the activation of lymphocytes, in addition to the critical recognition of the MHC/peptide complex.

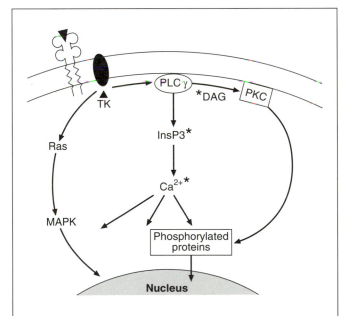

Fig. 3 Biochemical events leading to activation. Following interaction of the TCR with antigen, a number of biochemical events occur and second messengers (*) are produced which carry the signal generated at the cell surface to the nucleus mainly by phosphorylated proteins. These biochemical reactions occur within seconds/minutes of the receptor binding to the antigen. There is also evidence for activation of the ras GTPase and MAP kinase cascade. Similar events occur during early B cell activation. PLCγ, phospholipase C; DAG, diacylglycerol; InsP3, inositol 1, 4, 5 triphosphate; PKC, protein kinase C; TK, tyrosine kinases; MAPK, mitogen-activated protein kinase.

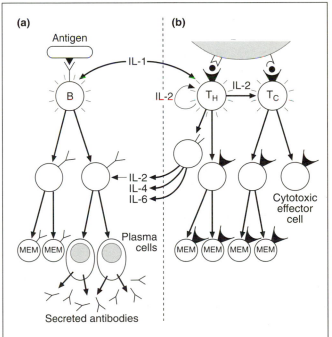

Fig. 4 Clonal selection. (a) Only B cells with receptors for the specific antigenic determinants of the microbe will be stimulated. In the presence of co-stimulatory cell signals, e.g. IL-1, the B cells proliferate and develop into plasma cells. The helper T cells produce various cytokines which are required for the production of both memory B cells and plasma cells. Note that all cells of the clone carry or contain antibodies of the same specificity as that of the original stimulated B cell. **(b)** Helper and cytotoxic T cell clones with memory cell members are produced in the same manner.

Adaptive Responses — Antibody

You will recall that following attack by a microbe, the natural immune system produces a rapid but not very specific response which may be totally adequate to dispose of the invader. In most cases, however, cells of the adaptive system come into contact with the antigens of the foreign invader, leading to adaptive immune responses. One important type of adaptive response is the antibody response.

The primary antibody response

Once induced, a primary antibody response has four phases (Fig. 1). During the initial *lag* period, prior to appearance of antibody in the serum, the antigen is localized and processed by various cells including macrophages and specific B cells; you remember that B cells responding to protein antigens require the help of T cells. The activated B lymphocytes proliferate and some differentiate into plasma cells during the *log* phase of the primary response. There then follows a *plateau* phase in which the antibody has bound to and removed free antigen (p. 35) so that the lymphocytes can no longer be stimulated. In addition, the plasma cells, being 'end' cells, simply die after they have carried out their function. Eventually the antigen is removed by the antibody via the various disposal mechanisms (p. 35) and the antibody response subsides leading to a *decline* of antibody in the serum.

The class switch

The first antibodies to be produced in a primary immune response are of the IgM class. IgG antibodies appear a few days later and follow the same phases as the IgM response. Figure 2 shows the cellular changes during the primary response by a single clone of B cells directed to a protein antigen, including the switch to IgG (p. 23).

Memory

In adaptive immune responses, the immune system 'remembers' that it has encountered antigen in the past. The characteristics of memory responses to subsequent contact with the same antigen are shown in Figure 3.

Many more specific cells of the B cell clone (memory cells) are present following the primary response (see Fig. 2), so more will be available to be stimulated by the antigen and more cells can differentiate into plasma cells. Thus, the secondary response is faster and bigger. As well as these *quantitative* changes in memory responses, there are *qualitative* changes in the antibody produced — class switching and affinity maturation. Memory antibody responses are highly dependent on T cells, little or no memory being seen in the absence of T cells.

Affinity maturation

Following antigenic stimulation and during the switch from IgM to IgG production, there is a high rate of **somatic mutations** in the genes coding for the antigen-binding region of the IgG molecule. Since these mutations are random, occasional cells with receptors able to bind more strongly to the antigen (i.e. with higher affinity) are produced and these are stimulated as the level of antigen drops due to disposal. Some mutations will give rise to Ig receptors which bind the antigen less well. These will not be stimulated by antigen and will therefore be of no use in a secondary response. The process of selection of memory cells occurs in the germinal centres of secondary follicles (Fig. 4).

Regulation

As well as the disposal of the antigen by antibodies (and therefore removal of the stimulus), active inhibition of antibody production occurs by a *negative feedback* mechanism involving IgG antibodies directly inhibiting specific B cells recognizing the antigen. This is mediated by IgG immune complexes and receptors on the surface of B cells for the Fc region of IgG (p. 23). Note: though these FcR are similar to those used by phagocytes, their function here is quite different.

Suppressor T cells are also thought to be important in regulating the antibody response by producing inhibitory cytokines.

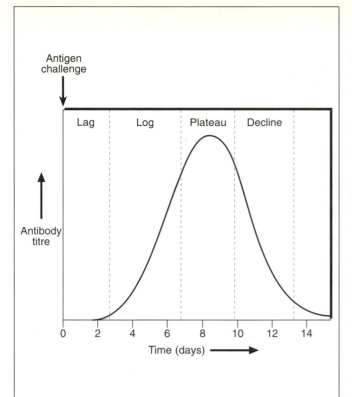

Fig. 1   **The four phases of the primary antibody response.** Note that the duration of the different phases and the absolute amount of antibody produced will vary from antigen to antigen and class to class of immunoglobulin (see Fig. 3).

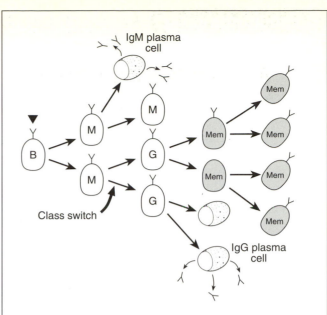

Fig. 2   **The cellular basis of the antibody response and switch from IgM to IgG.** Specific B cells of the IgM class are stimulated to divide and some of these differentiate into plasma cells secreting specific antibodies. During the proliferation phase, some of the IgM B cells 'switch' their antibody class to IgG. Some of these B cells also develop into IgG-secreting plasma cells but many become memory cells (MEM).

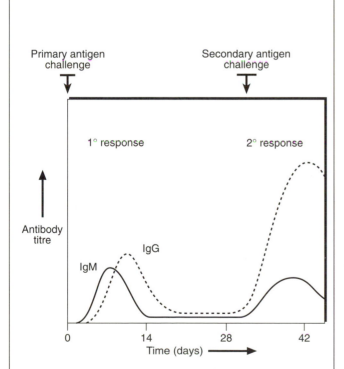

Fig. 3   **Memory responses to antigens.** Following restimulation with the antigen, the second antibody response shows a number of characteristics different from the primary response: (i) antibodies appear more rapidly; (ii) they reach higher levels; (iii) they are mainly of the IgG class; (iv) they are of higher average affinity.

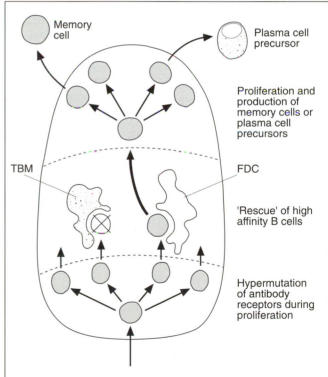

Fig. 4   **Cellular events in the follicular germinal centre.** An antigen-activated B cell enters the germinal centre, loses its surface antibody and proliferates. Somatic hypermutation occurs leading to cell suicide in some cells. Those cells with antibody receptors of high affinity are 'rescued' by recognizing antigen on the surface of follicular dendritic cells (FDC). The dead cells are phagocytosed by the tingible body macrophages (TBM). Rescued B cells will continue to divide and some become memory cells whilst others develop into plasma cell precursors; these leave the follicle and become plasma cells in the medulla of the lymph nodes or red pulp of the spleen.

Adaptive Responses — T Cells and Cell-mediated Immunity

We have already seen that T cells are necessary to help B cells to make most antibodies. Protection by antibodies is referred to as humoral immunity. **Cell-mediated immunity** or 'cellular' immunity is the term generally used to describe adaptive immune responses that do not involve antibodies, that is, involve T but not B cells.

The two major cell-mediated responses are quite distinct but they are both directed towards invading microbes which 'hide' inside cells of the body, i.e. intracellular microorganisms. They are carried out by separate subpopulations of T cell called **cytotoxic** and **helper.**

Cytotoxic T cells

T cells which carry the CD8 molecule recognize small peptides produced inside cells which bind to and are transported to the surface with the MHC class I molecules (p. 19). Such peptides are produced by **viruses** which might otherwise be invisible to the T cells. Once the T cell has recognized the MHC–peptide complex on the virus-infected cell through its antigen receptor, it develops into a cytotoxic cell which can then kill cells infected with the same virus (Fig. 1). The killing is brought about by various cytotoxic factors as described on page 35.

Helper T cells for cell-mediated immunity

We have already described the role of CD4 helper T cells in helping to activate B cells to make antibodies. You will remember that T cells which carry CD4 molecules recognize small peptides bound to MHC class II molecules. These peptides can also be derived from microbes living inside macrophages: for example, the tubercle bacillus and various fungal and protozoal parasites (see p. 39 for more about how they do this). On binding to the MHC–peptide complex on the macrophage surface, the T cell is stimulated to release cytokines, especially IFNγ, which activates the macrophage to be more effective in killing the intracellular microbe (Fig. 2). If this succeeds we say that the patient has recovered because of a cellular immune response; if it fails the patient will suffer a chronic infection and may even develop immunopathology.

Antigen processing and presentation

As you will have gathered from the above, which kind of T cell will be activated to function in cell-mediated immunity depends on whether the peptide is presented as a complex with MHC class I or II molecules. The two major pathways by which protein antigens are degraded (processed) and presented on the surface of antigen-presenting cells are shown in Figure 3. You should consult your cell biology textbook to remind yourself about endosomes, the Golgi apparatus and protein synthesis.

- **Endogenous antigen pathway.** Viruses living inside cells utilize the protein synthetic machinery of the cell to produce their own proteins. Viral peptides made in this way can bind to MHC class I molecules in Golgi-derived vesicles which then fuse with the external cell membrane, displaying MHC class I–peptide complexes to CD8 T cells (Fig. 3a). Here the T cell is being asked to *kill*.
- **Exogenous antigen pathway.** Exogenous antigens enter via endocytic vesicles which either (i) themselves contain MHC class II molecules and proteolytic enzymes or (ii) fuse with Golgi-derived vesicles carrying these proteins. The antigen is then degraded into peptides which associate with the MHC class II molecules to form an MHC–peptide complex which appears on the surface of the cell by reverse endocytosis. This is then available to interact with specific CD4 T cells (Fig. 3b). A similar process occurs in B lymphocytes that have bound to specific antigens through their antibody receptors. In both cases the T cell is being asked to *help*.

You can now see how the MHC molecules and T cells are a functional 'double act', the MHC molecules acting as a valuable device for allowing T cells to 'monitor' the inside of cells, where infectious organisms would otherwise be safely hidden away, and to take appropriate action. Remember that organisms which are not inside cells are vulnerable to attack by antibody (see pp. 23 & 35).

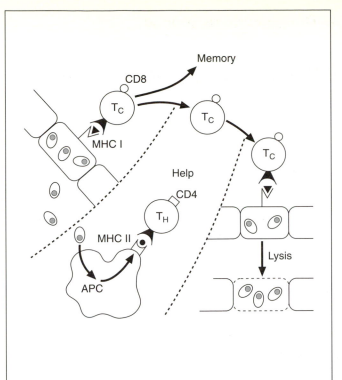

Fig. 1 Cytotoxic T cells. Viral particles released from infected cells are endocytosed by macrophages which process and present antigen to specific CD4 T cells. These help CD8 T cells, which recognize processed viral antigens with MHC class I molecules of infected cells, to develop into memory and effector cells. The CD8 T cells kill the cells infected with the same virus and secrete cytokines such as IFNγ which prevents infection of neighbouring cells by any released viable virions.

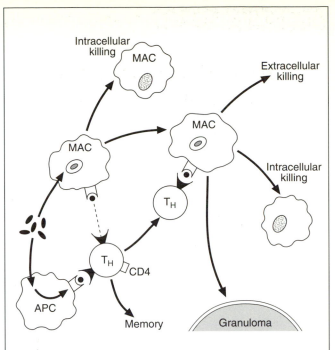

Fig. 2 Helper T cells in cell-mediated immunity. Macrophages may need help to kill their intracellular parasites. Infected or neighbouring macrophages display peptide antigens with MHC class II molecules. CD4 T cells recognize these and release cytokines which (i) enhance both the intracellular and extracellular killing of the microbes, e.g. IFNγ, and (ii) may help to form a granuloma if the macrophages contain non-degradeable materials such as tubercle bacilli or streptococcal cell walls.

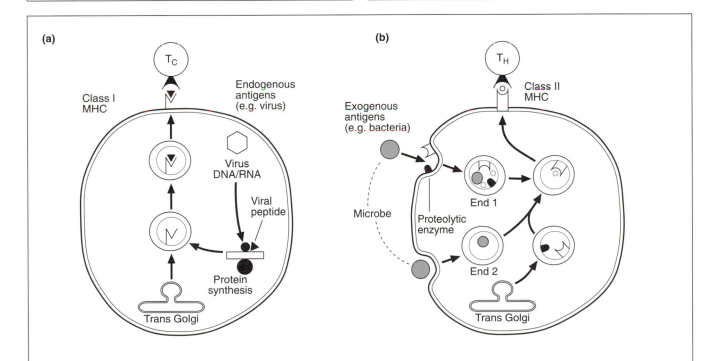

Fig. 3 Presentation of processed antigens to cytotoxic and helper T cells by different cells of the body. (a) Viruses can infect any nucleated cell of the body. Cells harbouring the viruses synthesize the viral proteins needed for replication and survival. Viral peptides are assembled on the ribosomes and are transported into Golgi-derived vesicles destined for the cell surface (reverse endocytosis). Newly assembled MHC class I molecules bind the viral peptides, usually in 9 amino acid stretches and the vesicles fuse with the cell surface. CD8 cytotoxic T cells that recognize the peptide-MHC class I complex can now kill the infected cell. (b) Larger microbes are taken into specialized antigen-presenting cells by phagocytosis. Their protein components are either degraded by cell membrane-derived proteolytic enzymes (e.g. cathepsin D) in the endosomes (END 1), or by enzymes made available by fusion of endosomes with newly 'budded' Golgi-derived vesicles containing these enzymes (END 2). Microbial peptides, 12 to 20 amino acids long, now bind to the MHC class II molecules replacing the small invariant chains already attached to them. These vesicles fuse with the cell surface to display peptide-MHC class II complexes to specific CD4 helper T cells.

Cytokines

A communication system

At this stage, you will have noticed that the immune system consists not just of cells acting individually, but of cells interacting with each other. Macrophages activate T cells, T cells activate macrophages, B cells and other T cells. In other words, it is an *integrated* system, as the endocrine and central nervous systems are; the main difference is that the cells of the immune system are not confined to one place but move around all over the body. These movements, and the interactions between the cells, are largely regulated by at least 20 (and probably far more) small protein molecules called **cytokines**.

Cytokines versus hormones

A rough analogy is to say that cytokines are the hormones of the immune system and there are certainly similarities: for instance, they have to bind to specific surface receptors in order to act on a cell, but the analogy is only partly valid, for the following reasons:

- Each cytokine can be made by more than one cell type, though macrophages and lymphocytes are the major source of most of them.
- Cytokines are much less specific than hormones and most of them have different effects on different cells, and even at different dose levels on the same cell. Contrariwise, quite different cytokines can have the same effect on a particular cell. At present everybody, including immunologists, finds this rather confusing.
- Cytokines frequently act together to increase, alter, or inhibit each other's activities. Thus most cells respond to a 'mix' of cytokines which may change from moment to moment. An example is shown in Figure 1.
- Though some cytokines undoubtedly act at a distance, their main effects are exerted between cells in close proximity. Cell biologists call this paracrine by contrast with the long-range endocrine signalling of the hormone system, where the cells themselves are not mobile.
- Finally it must be admitted that the definition of what is and what is not a cytokine is not totally precise. By general agreement, the molecules listed in Figure 2 are accepted as cytokines, but you will see that some of them have major effects on the haemopoietic as well as the immune system, and that you have already met some of them (the interferons) because of their anti-viral activity and others (the interleukins) because of their role in lymphocyte activation and the acute phase response. But there is no definition of a cytokine that would rule out the various growth factors (epidermal, nerve, etc.). Figure 3 gives an idea of the extraordinary ramifications of the cytokine 'network' in medicine.

Terminology

Originally, cytokines were named after their presumed function (interferon, tumour necrosis factor, T cell growth factor, etc.). But once it became obvious that each cytokine had several functions, an international committee (in 1978) decided that henceforth new cytokines should be called interleukins (i.e. 'between white cells') and numbered from IL-1 onwards. Many of the old names have, however, been retained, leading to the present inconsistent and confusing nomenclature.

Useful and harmful cytokines

Cytokines appear in several other parts of this book. The use of IFN in virus infection has already been mentioned, and both IFN and IL-2 are effective against certain cancers. The colony-stimulating factors have given impressive results in the treatment of bone marrow failure. But when produced excessively, some cytokines can cause unpleasant and dangerous side-effects, so they are also considered in the section on immunopathology. There is now a lot of interest in cytokine inhibitors and antagonists for dealing with such conditions, so it is likely that the pharmacy of the future will have on its shelves a range of both cytokines and anti-cytokines.

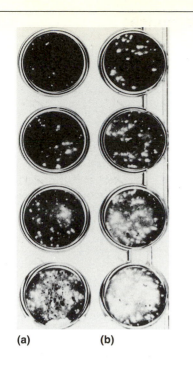

(a) **(b)**

Fig. 1 Synergy between cytokines. (a) TNFα secreted by macrophages plated out at four dilutions causes lysis of certain tumour cells. Here they are visible as unstained 'plaques' in a stained monolayer of tumour cells. **(b)** In the presence of IFNγ this anti-tumour activity is greatly enhanced. Unfortunately TNF does not have such striking anti-tumour activity in patients.

Cytokine	Molecular weight (kDa).	Principal source	Principal activities
IL-1	17	Macrophage	T, B cell activation, fever
IL-2	15–20	T cells	T, B cell proliferation
IL-3	14–30	T cells	Growth of many cell types
IL-4	15–19	T cells	B cell growth
IL-5	45	T cells	B cell, eosinophil growth
IL-6	26	T cells	B cell, liver stimulation
IL-7	25	T cells	Early B cell differentiation
IL-8	8.5	T cells	PMN, monocyte attraction
IL-9	32–39	T cells	Mast cell growth
IL-10	19	T cells	Inhibits other cytokines
IL-11	23	BM stroma	Haematopoiesis
IL-12	50	B cells	Stimulates T, NK cells
IL-13	12	T cells	Similar to IL-4; inhibits IFNγ
TGFβ	12.5 (× 2)	T cells	Inhibits other cytokines
IFNα	23	Most cells	Anti-viral; MHC I expression
IFNβ	23	Most cells	Anti-viral; MHC I expression
IFNγ	15–25	T, NK cells	Anti-viral, MHC II expression; macrophage activation
TNFα	17 (× 3)	Macrophage	Inflammation, fever (shock)
TNFβ (LT)	17 (× 3)	T cells	Inflammation, fever (shock)
GMCSF	18–24	Many cells	Myeloid cell growth
GCSF	20	Monocytes	Granulocyte growth
MCSF	22 (× 2)	Monocytes	Monocyte growth
*EPO	36	*Kidney	*Erythropoiesis

Fig. 2 The principal cytokines, showing their major cell(s) of origin and their major functions. IL, interleukin; TGF, transforming growth factor; IFN, interferon; TNF, tumour necrosis factor; LT, lymphotoxin; CSF, colony-stimulating factor (G, granulocyte; M, monocyte; GM, granulocyte/monocyte); EPO, erythropoietin. *Note: though EPO fits in here, it is not a typical cytokine, having a single origin and function, and acting only at a distance. There are also a number of other growth factors that some would include in the list of cytokines.

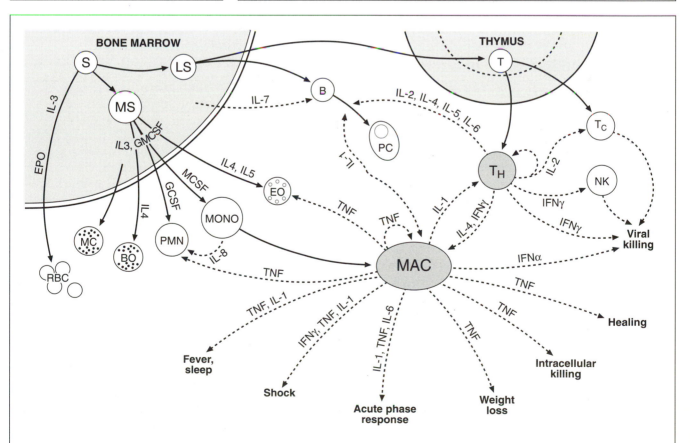

Fig. 3 The cytokine 'network', showing some of the cell differentiation pathways and interactions which are regulated by these molecules. Note the central role of T cells and macrophages in many protective as well as pathological responses. S, stem cell; MS, myeloid stem cell; MAC, macrophage; MC, mast cell; BO, basophil; EO, eosinophil; PC, plasma cell (the antibody-secreting cell); TC, cytotoxic T cell. For names of cytokines and more details on cell source, see Figure 2. (Adapted from Playfair J H L 1992 Immunology at a glance, 5th edn. Blackwell Scientific, Oxford.)

Disposal Mechanisms — Cytotoxicity

The 'eyes and teeth' of immunity

At the beginning of this book it was emphasized that the immune system has two duties in relation to infectious organisms: *recognition* and *disposal*. In everyday terms, it has 'eyes' and 'teeth'. We have discussed the eyes at some length (receptors, antibody, etc.) but mentioned the teeth only in passing (phagocytosis, complement, interferon, etc.) This is the time to review the mechanisms for destruction and disposal, looking in particular at those organisms against which they work best and also those that have learned how to resist them.

Most disposal is via natural mechanisms

The first point to make is that almost all the disposal mechanisms fall into the natural immune category, that is, they do not exhibit memory towards specific antigens. The one exception is the **cytotoxic T cell**, which is typically 'adaptive' in its specific recognition (via MHC molecules) and memory properties, but also carries out its own killing, using the same receptor through which it is activated. Because of this, its activities are restricted to targets carrying the appropriate MHC molecules, which in practice means virus-infected cells (Fig. 1), though there is also evidence for the killing of cells containing certain bacteria and even protozoa. By contrast, the **natural killer cell** specializes in killing cells that express little or no MHC molecules.

Intracellular killing: oxidative and non-oxidative

The killing mechanisms of phagocytic cells are of great interest (Fig. 2). Many of them derive from the stepwise reduction of atmospheric oxygen — the so-called 'respiratory' or 'oxygen burst' — during which some transient but very toxic **oxygen free radicals** are generated (Fig. 3). But phagocytes also contain numerous toxic proteins and other molecules, and one very simple molecule, **nitric oxide**, appears to be responsible for a good deal of killing, both intracellular and extracellular. In general, the killing mechanisms of PMN are better understood than those of macrophages.

The multiple roles of antibody

Finally, the scope of antibody in dealing with infection is worth summarizing here (Fig. 4). Essentially it is a recognition molecule, employed to bring together its specific target and non-specific disposal systems such as complement and/or phagocytic cells. Note, however, that getting a microbe into a phagocyte is only effective if the phagocyte can then kill it; many of the most successful parasites have sophisticated ways of avoiding being killed and indeed use the macrophage as a long-term residence: the tubercle bacillus is an example. There are also survival mechanisms against complement. In some cases antibody attaches its target to a cell which kills it without phagocytosing it; this is known as **antibody-dependent cell-mediated cytotoxicity** (**ADCC** for short) and it works with both macrophages and NK cells, but its actual role in infection is uncertain. Antibody can also act effectively on its own to physically block receptor–ligand interactions such as those required for toxins and viruses to enter cells. The familiar tetanus anti-toxin and the IgA antibody generated in the gut by the oral polio vaccine are good examples of this. As usual, the best guide to the real-life role of antibody is to look at patients who are deficient in it, and here we see that *defects in antibody production* have very much the same effect as defects in phagocytic cells, namely recurrent bacterial and fungal infection. This suggests that opsonization of bacteria, etc. for phagocytosis is, overall, its most important function and this is well illustrated by the sudden recovery of patients with pneumococcal pneumonia around day 7 — just the time it takes to make a good IgG response (this was in the days before antibiotics!). The antibody response to toxins is usually too slow to be of benefit, though of course a pre-existing level of anti-toxin can be life-saving, as happens with a second exposure to the same toxin or, better, in a patient who has been vaccinated.

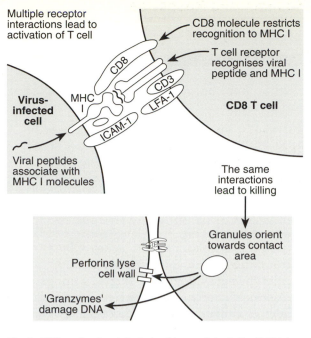

Fig. 1   Killing of a virus-infected cell by a cytotoxic T cell. This is a more detailed version of Figure 3, page 12, in which the contrast with NK cell killing is also emphasized.

Labels in Fig. 1:
Multiple receptor interactions lead to activation of T cell
CD8 molecule restricts recognition to MHC I
T cell receptor recognises viral peptide and MHC I
CD8 T cell
Virus-infected cell
MHC I, CD8, CD3, LFA-1, ICAM-1
Viral peptides associate with MHC I molecules
The same interactions lead to killing
Granules orient towards contact area
Perforins lyse cell wall
'Granzymes' damage DNA

Killing mechanism	Effective against
Oxidative killing	
Reactive oxygen intermediates (see Fig. 3)	Bacteria, fungi, some protozoa
Non-oxidative killing	
Reactive nitrogen intermediates (nitric oxide)	Bacteria, fungi, some protozoa
Lysozyme	Bacterial cell wall (Gram +)
Cationic 'defensins'	Bacteria, viruses
Bacterial permeability increasing factor	Bacterial LPS (Gram −)
Lactoferrin	Bacterial iron supplies
Vitamin B12 binding protein	Bacteria
Vitamin C + copper	Bacteria
Elastase	Bacteria
Cathepsin G	Bacteria, fungi
Major basic protein ⎫ Eosinophil cationic proteins ⎬	Worms ? (eosinophils only)
Cathepsins B, D	Mainly digestive
Proteases	Mainly digestive
β Glucuronidase	Mainly digestive
Collagenase	Mainly digestive
Gelatinase	Mainly digestive

Fig. 2   Killing and digestion in granulocytes. The granules of PMN contain a wide range of systems for killing and digesting microbes, notably bacteria. Eosinophils also have their own granule contents. Many of the above are also present in monocytes and macrophages, but here their role is not so well understood.

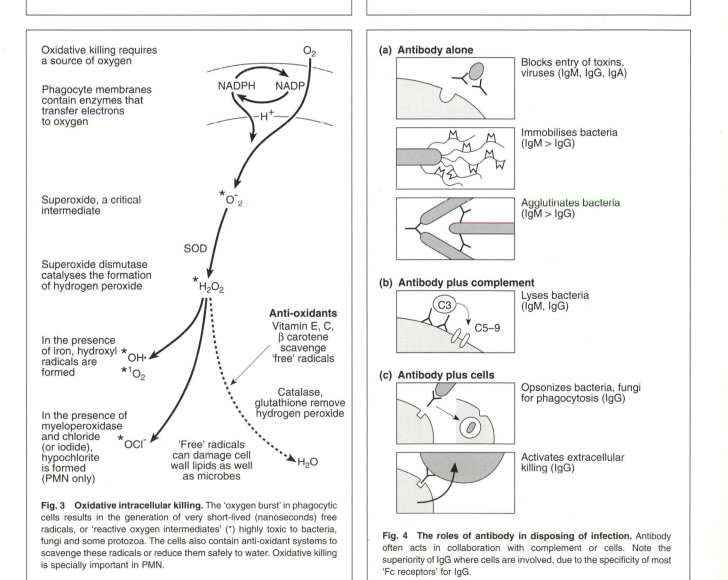

Fig. 3   Oxidative intracellular killing. The 'oxygen burst' in phagocytic cells results in the generation of very short-lived (nanoseconds) free radicals, or 'reactive oxygen intermediates' (*) highly toxic to bacteria, fungi and some protozoa. The cells also contain anti-oxidant systems to scavenge these radicals or reduce them safely to water. Oxidative killing is specially important in PMN.

Labels in Fig. 3:
Oxidative killing requires a source of oxygen
Phagocyte membranes contain enzymes that transfer electrons to oxygen
O_2, NADPH, NADP, $-H^+$
Superoxide, a critical intermediate — $*O_2^-$
SOD
Superoxide dismutase catalyses the formation of hydrogen peroxide — $*H_2O_2$
In the presence of iron, hydroxyl radicals are formed — $*OH\cdot$ $*{}^1O_2$
In the presence of myeloperoxidase and chloride (or iodide), hypochlorite is formed (PMN only) — $*OCl^-$
Anti-oxidants — Vitamin E, C, β carotene scavenge 'free' radicals
Catalase, glutathione remove hydrogen peroxide
'Free' radicals can damage cell wall lipids as well as microbes — H_2O

Fig. 4   The roles of antibody in disposing of infection. Antibody often acts in collaboration with complement or cells. Note the superiority of IgG where cells are involved, due to the specificity of most 'Fc receptors' for IgG.

Labels in Fig. 4:
(a) Antibody alone
Blocks entry of toxins, viruses (IgM, IgG, IgA)
Immobilises bacteria (IgM > IgG)
Agglutinates bacteria (IgM > IgG)
(b) Antibody plus complement
C3, C5–9
Lyses bacteria (IgM, IgG)
(c) Antibody plus cells
Opsonizes bacteria, fungi for phagocytosis (IgG)
Activates extracellular killing (IgG)

36

Immunity to Infection — Host Defence Mechanisms

Parasite and host: well-matched opponents

A variety of microorganisms parasitize the human body and some of them cause disease. However, this is not necessarily their main aim, which is to get in, live at our expense and (usually) be transmitted to another individual. The aim of the immune system is to kill or dislodge them, and in most infections the result is a battle between two fairly well-matched forces (Fig. 1). Parasitism is represented in six classes of organisms, as follows:

- **Viruses** can only replicate within cells, have DNA or RNA genomes, are only visible in the electron microscope (Fig. 2) and enter by specific receptors (Fig. 3). Examples: most of the common childhood infections (measles, mumps, rubella, chickenpox), also hepatitis, herpes. Immunity is usually good, but there are important exceptions (colds, flu, HIV).
- **Bacteria** are single procaryotic cells, visible under the light microscope (Fig. 4) with walls and often capsules, flagella, pili, etc. They may live extracellularly (e.g. staphylococci; streptococci) or intracellularly (e.g. the tubercle bacillus). Other examples: typhoid, whooping cough. Some secrete powerful toxins, examples: tetanus, diphtheria, cholera, staphylococci. Immunity varies from good to very poor.
- **Fungi** (Fig. 5) are eucaryotes (more similar to mammalian cells) but resemble bacteria from the immunological point of view. Examples: candida (yeast), histoplasma, cryptococci.
- **Protozoa** (Fig. 6) are again eucaryotes but with highly developed mechanisms for escaping the immune system; they only induce partial immunity at best. Examples: malaria, amoeba, trypanosomes, leishmania, toxoplasma.
- **Helminths** (worms) are multicellular organisms, far too large to be intracellular (Fig. 7) but may inhabit the tissues or the intestine. Immunity is usually fairly ineffective. Examples: tapeworms, hookworm, schistosome, filaria. Unlike other parasites, they do not replicate in the human body.
- **Ectoparasites** (i.e. outside the body). Examples: ticks, lice. No effective immunity.

Note: plenty of bacteria, fungi, protozoa and worms are not parasitic but live free in soil, water, etc. For further details of classification, life cycles, etc. consult your microbiology text-books.

Effective immunity

Many parasites are rapidly dealt with by natural immune mechanisms and never get a foothold. By definition, these do not cause disease. With the ones that do, the point to remember is that the kind of immune mechanism likely to be effective depends largely on where the parasite is situated, and particularly whether it is inside a cell or free in the extracellular compartments.

- **Extracellular parasites** are usually susceptible to antibody, since they cannot easily avoid their antigens being 'seen' by B cells nor escape from antibody binding to their surface. This applies especially to extracellular bacteria, but also to viruses in, e.g. the blood. See the previous page for details of how antibody can protect against toxins and opsonize for phagocytosis or lysis by complement; the latter operates mainly against neisseria (meningococci, gonococci). See also the following page for the cunning strategies some parasites have evolved to escape recognition and/or disposal.
- **Intracellular parasites** usually require a response by T cells: either the CD8 cytotoxic type (for viruses) or the CD4 helper type that secrete cytokines and activate killing within macrophages (for tubercle, leishmania, etc.). Antibody does not normally affect a parasite once it is in a cell. The entire MHC system can be regarded as a way for parasitized cells to inform T cells of what is inside them and to summon help in dealing with it. Here again, some parasites can sabotage the system (see p. 39).

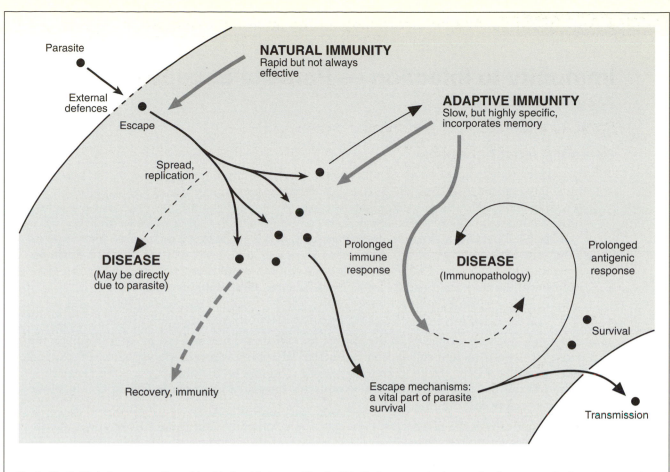

Fig. 1 The battle between parasite and host is fought at several levels. Note the importance for the parasite of escape mechanisms. Note also that disease — that is, pathology, symptoms — can be due to the parasite itself or to an excessive immune response.

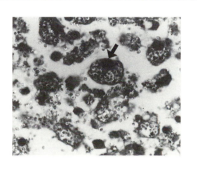

Fig. 2 Human wart virus.

Virus	Receptor
Epstein–Barr	B cell complement receptor
HIV	T cell, macrophage CD4
Rhinovirus	Adhesion molecule ICAM-1
Rabies	Acetylcholine receptor
Vaccinia	Epidermal growth factor receptor
Influenza	Glycophorin A (also on red cells)
Reovirus	β adrenergic hormone receptor

Fig. 3 Viral binding receptors. All viruses need to bind to a specific cell surface molecule ('receptor') in order to get in, but only some of these have been identified. This binding is vulnerable to blocking by antibody, but in some cases antibody can also help the virus to enter.

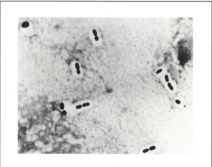

Fig. 4 Bacteria. Negative staining (with Indian ink) of these pneumococci reveals the gelatinous polysaccharide capsule, a major anti-phagocytic protective device.

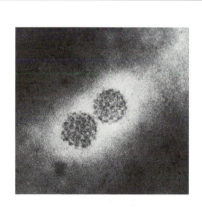

Fig. 5 Fungal infection. Bone marrow from a case of histoplasmosis, showing macrophages (nuclei arrowed) stuffed with fungal particles.

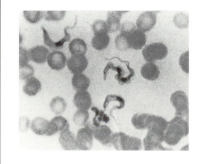

Fig. 6 Trypanosomes from a case of sleeping sickness. These protozoa live free in the blood — a most unusual habitat for any organism.

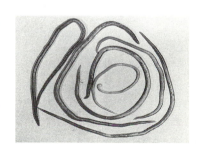

Fig. 7 Helminth infestation. The round-worm Ascaris can grow up to 30 cm in length. Like most parasitic worms, they are virtually out of reach of the immune system because of their size and toughness.

38

Immunity to Infection — Parasite Escape Mechanisms

Parasites must fight back

To survive the powerful forces of natural and adaptive immunity ranged against it, a parasite must have one or several survival strategies. By definition, this is true of all successful parasites, which includes all those of medical interest. We need to understand these survival strategies in order to understand why some infections become chronic, why some vaccines do not work, etc.

Think of a parasite as a spy in enemy territory, in danger of being recognized and disposed of. How is he to survive? There are many ways: to stay in hiding, to go out in disguise, to shoot anyone who comes near. Parasites use all these strategies and more, tailoring their strategy to the immune attack they are most in danger from. Some examples are given below.

Avoiding phagocytosis (Fig. 1). This is particularly important for bacteria such as staphylococci and streptococci that are easily killed in phagocytes. The gelatinous polysaccharide capsule effectively prevents contact with the phagocyte; capsulated bacteria can be up to a million times more virulent than identical but non-capsulated strains. However, antibody against the capsule can cancel this advantage by linking up with Fc receptors on the phagocyte. Staphylococci secrete toxins that kill phagocytes and a molecule (protein A) that neutralizes antibody; other bacteria secrete enzymes that destroy IgA.

Avoiding death in the phagocyte. Here it is a question of avoiding attack by oxygen radicals and the contents of lysosomes. Figure 2 shows a variety of strategies and you will see that the parasites responsible, mostly bacteria or protozoa, account for some of the most chronic and intractable infections.

Avoiding complement (Fig. 3). Anything that stops the C3bBb complex contacting the microbial wall can prevent the alternative pathway being activated; this includes capsules, long polysaccharide chains, non-complement-activating antibodies. Some protozoa can actually expel the membrane attack complex, somewhat like a 'self-sealing' bicycle tyre.

Avoiding interferon and other cytokines (see Fig. 4). A sensible strategy for viruses.

Avoiding recognition by lymphocytes (Fig. 5). A very large field. Parasite strategies to avoid recognition essentially fall into three categories:

- *Concealment.* Parts of the body are not regularly visited by lymphocytes (skin surface, excretory glands, gut contents, brain, testis, placenta); here the parasite is safe from recognition. Some, especially worms, take up host molecules and become 'invisible', while others have learned to 'mimic' host antigens, though this more often leads to autoimmunity (e.g. streptococci in the myocardium) than to parasite survival.
- *Antigenic variation.* The well-known fact that immunity to influenza acquired one year does not work the next year is explained by the virus's ability to mutate its surface antigens and/or recombine parts of its genome with other (animal) viruses. HIV is another virus that can vary its receptor-binding (gp120) antigen extensively. African trypanosomes carry antigen variation even further; their genome contains DNA coding for about 1000 totally different possible surface coat proteins that can be switched on and off rapidly. The unfortunate host is obliged to make new primary antibody responses at weekly intervals — an impossible task to keep up.
- *Immunosuppression.* The power of HIV to suppress T cell immunity is all too familiar, but similar effects are seen with many protozoa (trypanosomes, malaria), bacteria (TB) and, more transiently, other viruses (measles). Some parasite-derived molecules go to the opposite extreme and activate practically *all* lymphocytes, which effectively means that specific responses are 'crowded out'.

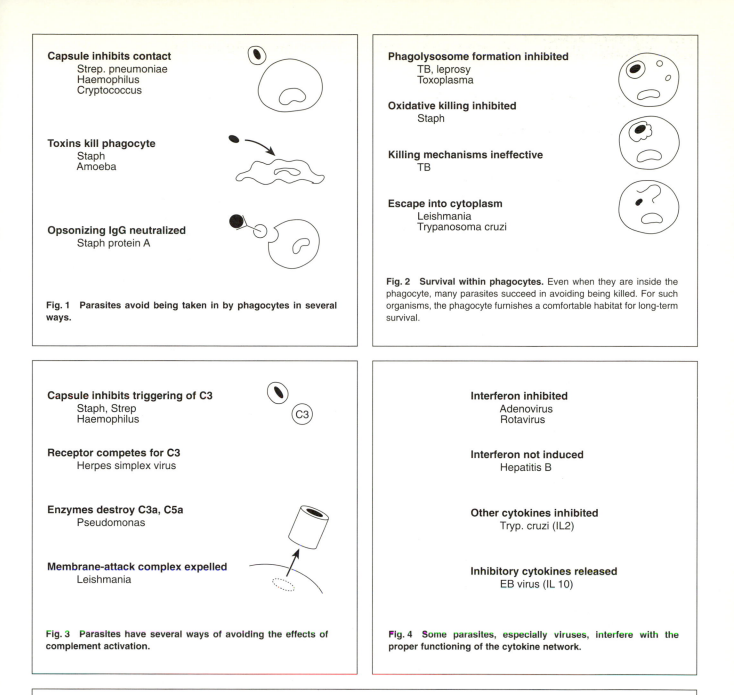

Capsule inhibits contact
Strep. pneumoniae
Haemophilus
Cryptococcus

Toxins kill phagocyte
Staph
Amoeba

Opsonizing IgG neutralized
Staph protein A

Fig. 1 Parasites avoid being taken in by phagocytes in several ways.

Phagolysosome formation inhibited
TB, leprosy
Toxoplasma

Oxidative killing inhibited
Staph

Killing mechanisms ineffective
TB

Escape into cytoplasm
Leishmania
Trypanosoma cruzi

Fig. 2 **Survival within phagocytes.** Even when they are inside the phagocyte, many parasites succeed in avoiding being killed. For such organisms, the phagocyte furnishes a comfortable habitat for long-term survival.

Capsule inhibits triggering of C3
Staph, Strep
Haemophilus

Receptor competes for C3
Herpes simplex virus

Enzymes destroy C3a, C5a
Pseudomonas

Membrane-attack complex expelled
Leishmania

Fig. 3 Parasites have several ways of avoiding the effects of complement activation.

Interferon inhibited
Adenovirus
Rotavirus

Interferon not induced
Hepatitis B

Other cytokines inhibited
Tryp. cruzi (IL2)

Inhibitory cytokines released
EB virus (IL 10)

Fig. 4 **Some parasites, especially viruses, interfere with the proper functioning of the cytokine network.**

Concealment of antigens	Antigenic variation and diversity	Immunosuppression
Virus latent Herpes simplex, varicella-zoster	**Mutation** Influenza H and N antigens, HIV Many other viruses, bacteria, etc.	**Infection of lymphocytes** HIV (T) Measles (T) Cytomegalovirus (T) EB virus (B)
MHC expression inhibited Adenovirus	**Recombination** Influenza (with animal viruses) Neisseria	**Interference with cytokines (see Fig. 4)**
Privileged site DNA (retroviruses) Skin surface, intestine Hydatid worm in cyst	**Gene switching** African trypanosomes Borreliae	**Polyclonal lymphocyte activation** Gram-negative bacterial LPS (B) Staphylococcal enterotoxins (T)
Uptake of host antigen Schistosome worm Cytomegalovirus	**Serological diversity ('polymorphism')** Adenovirus, rhinovirus Enteroviruses *Strep. pneumoniae* *Salmonella typhi* Plasmodium (malaria)	**Macrophage over-activation (?)** Malaria
Mimicry of host antigens Streptococci (myocardium) Klebsiellae (HLA B27) Spirochaete (cardiolipin)		

Fig. 5 **Avoidance of adaptive immunity.** This is essentially a problem of avoiding *recognition* by lymphocyte receptors, since the disposal mechanisms are mostly those dealt with in Figures 1–4. Note that antigenic diversity is simply the result of extensive antigenic variation in the past.

40

Tutorial 3

You have now been exposed to all the information necessary for the understanding of the normal working of the immune system, a position roughly equivalent to the end of the first year of most medical or science courses. You should therefore be able to answer the questions below. Specimen answers opposite.

Questions

1. What stimuli are required for a lymphocyte to proliferate into a clone?

2. What advantage is there in the fact that T cells recognize MHC as well as foreign peptides?

3. Name three differences between typical primary and secondary antibody responses.

4. In what way are cytokines (a) similar to, (b) different from hormones ?

5. Name three activities of gamma interferon.

6. How do NK cells and cytotoxic T cells differ in killing virus-infected cells?

7. Why do individual B cells switch constant but not variable genes?

8. Explain the term clonal selection.

9. Why do normal immune responses not go on for ever ?

10. Name three ways in which a microorganism can avoid being killed by a phagocytic cell. What may be the consequence?

Further reading

Virtually every immunology textbook covers adaptive responses very adequately. Consult 'Milestones in immunology' to see the gradual evolution of the clonal selection theory. Here is some extra reading that will amplify the last four topics in this section.

Meager A 1990 Cytokines. Open University Press, Milton Keynes, UK, 291 pp. Of the numerous books on cytokines, this is on the whole the easiest to read and most informative. There are frequent meetings on individual cytokines (IFN, TNF, IL-2, etc.) which are later published as books (usually expensive !).

Hamblin A S 1988 Lymphokines. IRL Press, Oxford. A good short book on cytokines, written in simple language and well-referenced.

Mims C A 1987 The pathogenesis of infectious disease, 3rd edn. Academic Press, London, 342 pp. The only modest-sized book that tackles the interface between microbiology, immunology and pathology. Extremely readable, it gives a vivid feeling of the 'battle' between host and parasite.

Mims C A, Playfair J H L, Roitt I M, Wakelin D, Williams R 1993 Medical microbiology. Mosby, London. A microbiology textbook with more immunology than usual and, again, an emphasis on the battle. The hundreds of colour illustrations are available as a slide atlas.

Answers

1. Interaction between antigen and antigen-specific receptors on the lymphocyte: for B cells, antibody–antigen; for T cells, T cell receptor-MHC + peptide and MHC-CD4 or CD8. Co-stimulatory signals: cytokines (mainly interleukins).

2. It ensures that T cells only interact with cells to which they can do something useful. Thus, any cell infected with a virus can be killed (via CD8-MHC class I) and any cell harbouring a persistent bacterium, fungus, protozoan, etc. can be activated (via CD4-MHC class II). It would be pointless for T cells to recognize isolated microorganisms since they have no way of dealing directly with them.

3. Secondary responses start sooner, reach higher levels, last longer, contain more IgG, contain more high-affinity antibody.

4. Similar in acting as chemical messengers between cells, binding to surface receptors; different in having numerous and overlapping functions, acting mainly synergistically and at close range. Note also that cytokines are proteins and fairly similar in size (15–50 kDa) whereas hormones vary greatly (hydrocortisone 360, thyroxine 800, insulin 6000, parathyroid hormone 10 kDa).

5. Anti-viral (like all interferons); activates macrophages, NK cells, PMN; enhances MHC class II expression; stimulates B cells (but may also inhibit them); synergizes with TNF.

6. Chiefly at the recognition stage. Cytotoxic T cells recognize specific viral peptides in the groove of MHC class I molecules; NK cells recognize unidentified carbohydrates and also the Fc portion of IgG, if the latter is bound to the target cell. Once recognition has occurred, the cytotoxic mechanisms of the two types of cell are thought to be similar.

7. By switching C genes, a B cell can produce antibody with a different biological usefulness, e.g. switching from IgM to IgG allows the antibody to bind to Fc receptors on phagocytes. If a B cell switched V genes, it would produce antibody of a different specificity which would have no relevance to the inducing antigen and would probably be useless at that particular moment. Note, however, that small changes in the V region produced by mutation may occasionally lead to a better-fitting antibody, that is, antibody of a higher affinity; this is called **affinity maturation**.

8. Selection refers to the effect of a particular antigen in selecting out of millions of lymphocytes those few that recognize it. Clonal refers to the subsequent proliferation of these selected lymphocytes into a population of identical cells (a clone) large enough to produce an effective response.

9. In the great majority of cases, elimination of the antigen removes the stimulus to the B and T cells, so that these are no longer driven to proliferate and function. Antibody can also limit its own production via the inhibitory effect of immune complexes on B cells. In addition, there are two more controversial mechanisms, thought to be especially important where antigen elimination is impossible, for example where the response is against a self-antigen or some parasite such as a worm that cannot be dislodged; both suppressor T cells and anti-antibodies (anti-idiotype) have been found in such situations.

10. By preventing attachment (capsule), by killing the phagocyte (toxin), by inhibiting phagosome–lysosome fusion, by destroying oxygen radicals, by escaping into the cytoplasm. Prevention of phagocytosis may result in difficulty in containing the infection (e.g. a staphylococcal abscess); survival in macrophages may result in chronic infection with a strong likelihood of immunopathology. How this works is described in the next section.

Acute and Chronic Inflammation

Chronic usually follows acute

First, look back at page 11 to be reminded that acute inflammation is the normal response to most forms of injury or infection. Normally, one would expect it to last only a matter of days or at most weeks, since disposal of infectious organisms and repair of tissue damage will gradually remove the inflammatory stimulus. Sometimes, however, this does not happen and inflammation becomes *chronic*. A wound may not heal because there are foreign bodies in it. Infection may continue because neither the immune system nor the doctor can stop it; this is especially common with those intracellular organisms that resist being killed by macrophages (p. 39). Alternatively, the signs of chronic inflammation may be present without any obvious cause and without the usual acute inflammatory stage; several important diseases fall into this category.

The macrophage in centre stage — again!

Just as PMN, mast cells and complement are the main actors in acute inflammation, chronic inflammation chiefly reflects the actions, or failure to act, of macrophages. They may be there in their role as scavengers, engulfing small particles or summoning more macrophages to surround large ones and form a **granuloma** (Fig. 1). If the particles cannot be degraded, such a granuloma may persist virtually for ever. Macrophages may coalesce to form multinucleated **giant cells** (Fig. 2) which have an increased degradative ability. Sometimes the foreign material is not only undegradeable but toxic, and in such cases new macrophages may have to be recruited continuously to contain the danger.

Immunological and non-immunological granulomas

All the events described above can occur in the absence of any specific recognition of the foreign material by lymphocytes. But when the foreign material takes the form of an infectious microorganism, lymphocytes usually are involved and they can substantially influence the course of the inflammation. Histologically one sees lymphocytes, particularly T cells, among the macrophages, and often also eosinophils and specialized secretory macrophages called **epithelioid cells** (Fig. 3). Several T cell-derived cytokines play a role in attracting, immobilizing and activating other cells — a typical cell-mediated response — and, because of the 'memory' properties of the lymphocytes, the lesions may grow progressively in size to the point where they can seriously affect organ function (Figs 4, 5 & 6). At this stage we are clearly in the realm of **immunopathology**.

To react or not to react?

Immunological granuloma formation illustrates vividly the dilemma of chronic infection: whether to keep up a vigorous cell-mediated response and possibly end up with organ damage or to allow the invading organism to flourish unchecked. Often both courses are bad; for example in leprosy, both the tuberculoid (strong CMI) and the lepromatous form (no CMI) are extremely unpleasant for the patient. In the same way, a patient with schistosomiasis who did not make granulomas round the eggs would die of liver failure due to the highly toxic egg secretions. Sometimes you cannot win.

Amyloidosis and the immune response

The deposition of eosinophilic birefringent fibrils recognized by histopathologists as **amyloid** can be the result of immune processes in two quite separate ways: (1) overproduction of immunoglobulins (e.g. in myelomatosis) whose light chains (mainly λ) form into β-pleated sheets in skin, joints, heart, etc; (2) deposition of structurally similar material derived from the acute-phase reactant serum amyloid A protein during prolonged chronic inflammatory responses (e.g. TB) in liver, spleen, kidneys, adrenals, etc.

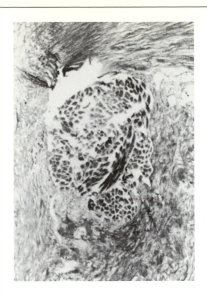

Fig. 1 A small granuloma formed around a piece of surgical suture. Such lesions can persist for years without significant changes in size. If the foreign material is toxic (e.g. silica), macrophages will be killed and continuously replaced — the 'high turnover' granuloma.

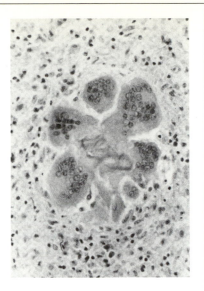

Fig. 2 Multinucleated giant cells. Also called polykaryons, these are produced by fusion of the membranes of several macrophages. They contain raised levels of enzymes and appear to have increased digestive ability.

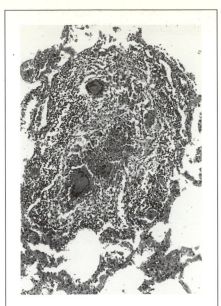

Fig. 3 A typical tuberculous granuloma, containing giant cells and numerous epithelioid cells, with central necrosis ('caseation'). The caseation is probably due to cell destruction by macrophage enzymes, but does not occur in otherwise similar granulomas, e.g. in sarcoidosis.

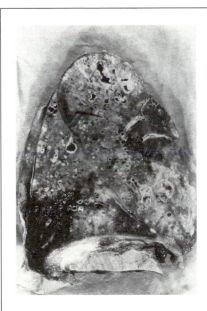

Fig. 4 A lung from an advanced case of tuberculosis. Extensive caseation and cavitation have occurred, especially towards the apex. The best result that could be hoped for at this stage would be healing with fibrosis, but clearly some lung function would be lost.

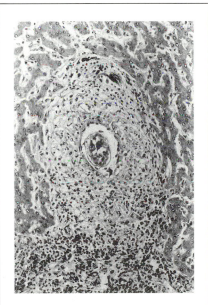

Fig. 5 A granuloma surrounding an egg of the liver fluke *Schistosoma mansoni*, which has lodged in a small portal vein. Note the healthy state of the liver parenchyma, protected by the granuloma from the highly toxic enzymes secreted by the egg.

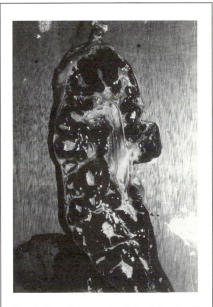

Fig. 6 Massive periportal ('pipestem') fibrosis from the coalescence of millions of *S. mansoni* egg granulomas. This eventually leads to portal hypertension with hepatosplenomegaly and often fatal haematemesis from ruptured oesophageal varices.

Hypersensitivity

Some confusing terminology

The contribution of T cells to granuloma formation in, for example, TB (p. 43) is a case of adaptive immunity (the T cell) collaborating with natural immunity (the macrophage). The main objective is to protect the host, but in the process considerable tissue damage can be done. When discussing this damage, we speak of **immunopathology**, but when thinking about the role of the immune system, the term **hypersensitivity** is also used: the implication being that the host, through the development of adaptive immunity, has become 'too sensitive' to the foreign material (i.e. the tubercle bacillus) for his own good. There are several ways in which this can happen and, ironically, the antigens involved are not always particularly virulent (e.g. allergy to animal fur or pollen).

Skin testing

The existence of hypersensitivity has been known for almost 100 years, though the understanding of what caused it had to wait until the immune response itself was understood. The early workers knew that injecting foreign material into the skin of people who have already been exposed to the same material could induce visible reactions of various kinds. Swelling and redness that came up within minutes was called **immediate hypersensitivity** and it was soon found that harmless substances like pollen and horse serum could cause this; we now know that they denote the presence of antibody, especially IgE. If the reaction took 2–3 days, it was called **delayed hypersensitivity** and, because this was first noted in tuberculosis, it was also known as bacterial allergy; this was later shown to be a sign of T cell immunity. Immediate and delayed skin tests are still in use, the first to detect the offending antigen in patients with hay fever, etc., the latter to evaluate cell-mediated immune status in TB and similar diseases (see Fig. 1).

A rational classification

The British immunologists Philip Gell and Robin Coombs tackled the problem of nomenclature of hypersensitivity reactions and produced the Gell and Coombs classification, which is still widely used. They defined *four types* of hypersensitivity, of which the T cell-granuloma response described above was type IV, types I – III being dependent on antibody rather than T cells. A major virtue of this new nomenclature was to distinguish between three quite different ways in which antibody could lead to pathology: namely via IgE (allergies), IgG (cytotoxicity) and antibody–antigen complexes (vascular damage). Figure 1 sets out the details, together with some small modifications that have had to be made more recently.

Unfortunately the terminology is still not perfect; for example, the activation of macrophages to kill an intracellular parasite and the destruction of a lung by fibrosed granulomas are both often loosely referred to as delayed hypersensitivity although this term originally meant just the skin test. 'Type IV hypersensitivity' would be one step nearer, but the best solution is to understand the actual immunological and pathological mechanisms involved — which T cells, which cytokines, which macrophages, which other cells, etc. Once these are clear in the mind, it does not matter so much which term is used to describe the phenomenon.

Natural immunity can damage your health too

Recently it has become apparent that macrophages can cause pathology even without help from T cells, the most striking example being when they are stimulated by **lipopolysaccharide** (**LPS**) from Gram-negative bacteria (p. 49). Direct stimulation of PMN and activation of complement can also lead to pathology. There is no generally accepted terminology yet for this type of reaction, but it is not usually included under the heading of hypersensitivity.

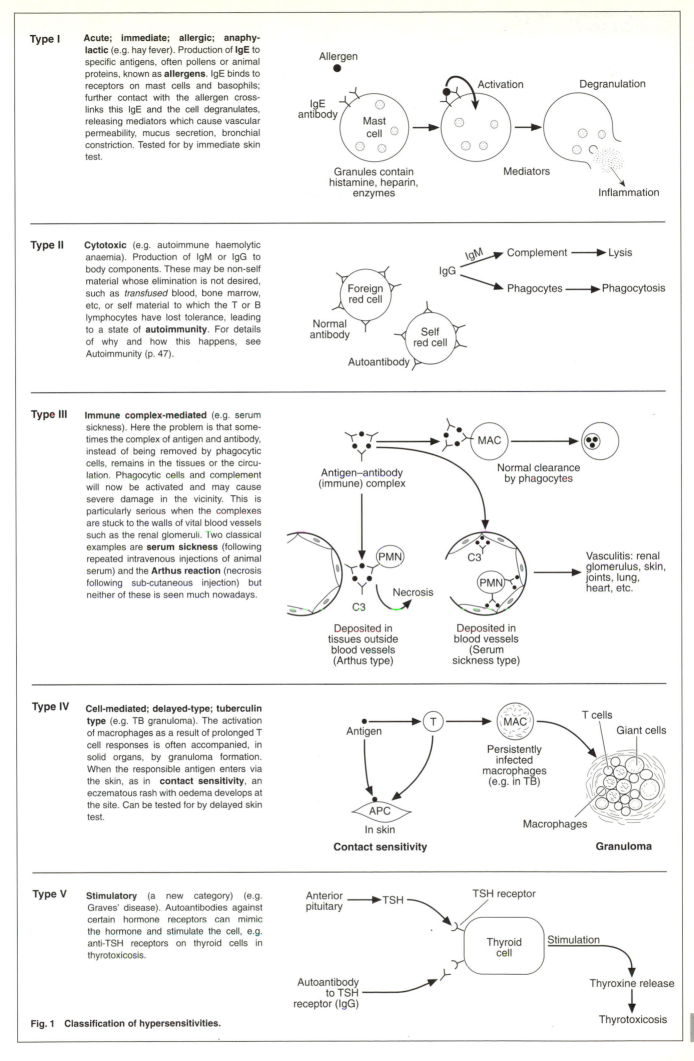

Type I **Acute; immediate; allergic; anaphylactic** (e.g. hay fever). Production of **IgE** to specific antigens, often pollens or animal proteins, known as **allergens**. IgE binds to receptors on mast cells and basophils; further contact with the allergen cross-links this IgE and the cell degranulates, releasing mediators which cause vascular permeability, mucus secretion, bronchial constriction. Tested for by immediate skin test.

Type II **Cytotoxic** (e.g. autoimmune haemolytic anaemia). Production of IgM or IgG to body components. These may be non-self material whose elimination is not desired, such as *transfused* blood, bone marrow, etc, or self material to which the T or B lymphocytes have lost tolerance, leading to a state of **autoimmunity**. For details of why and how this happens, see Autoimmunity (p. 47).

Type III **Immune complex-mediated** (e.g. serum sickness). Here the problem is that sometimes the complex of antigen and antibody, instead of being removed by phagocytic cells, remains in the tissues or the circulation. Phagocytic cells and complement will now be activated and may cause severe damage in the vicinity. This is particularly serious when the complexes are stuck to the walls of vital blood vessels such as the renal glomeruli. Two classical examples are **serum sickness** (following repeated intravenous injections of animal serum) and the **Arthus reaction** (necrosis following sub-cutaneous injection) but neither of these is seen much nowadays.

Type IV **Cell-mediated; delayed-type; tuberculin type** (e.g. TB granuloma). The activation of macrophages as a result of prolonged T cell responses is often accompanied, in solid organs, by granuloma formation. When the responsible antigen enters via the skin, as in **contact sensitivity**, an eczematous rash with oedema develops at the site. Can be tested for by delayed skin test.

Type V **Stimulatory** (a new category) (e.g. Graves' disease). Autoantibodies against certain hormone receptors can mimic the hormone and stimulate the cell, e.g. anti-TSH receptors on thyroid cells in thyrotoxicosis.

Fig. 1 Classification of hypersensitivities.

46

Autoimmunity

Autoimmunity is the result of a breakdown in self-tolerance leading to cellular and/or antibody responses to body components. In many cases, this leads to **autoimmune diseases** which affect up to 7% of the population.

Spectrum of autoimmune disease

Autoimmune diseases may affect many organs of the body, but conventionally they are classified into either **organ** or **non-organ specific**, according to whether the autoimmune response affects one major target organ (or tissue), or several organs of the body. This distinction is not perfect and in polyendocrine autoimmune disease and primary biliary cirrhosis more than one gland is affected (pp. 61–64). Autoimmune diseases and their target antigens are listed in Figure 1.

Organ-specific autoimmune diseases

Hashimoto's disease is a classical example of an organ-specific disorder in which the thyroid undergoes destructive infiltration by mononuclear cells and thyroid autoantibodies are produced (Fig. 1). The mechanisms for tissue damage appear to be different for the two major kinds of autoimmune diseases and in organ-specific disease this is mediated through *type II, type IV* or *type V* hypersensitivities (p. 45). For example, in myasthenia gravis (MG), autoantibodies to acetylcholine receptors block transmission of nerve impulses at motor end plate junctions. Occasionally, transient autoimmune disease is found in newborn babies of mothers with MG, due to immunoglobulin transfer across the placenta. A similar process can occur in babies born to mothers with Graves' disease who have autoantibodies directed to the thyroid-stimulating hormone (TSH) receptors (type V). Type IV hypersensitivity is thought to play an important role in tissue damage of the islet cells in insulin-dependent diabetes mellitus.

Non-organ specific autoimmune diseases

Some of the important non-organ specific autoimmune diseases are shown in Figure 1. Here, the autoantigens are not limited to specific organs but are common to cells in different organs and tissues. Unlike organ-specific disease, the major mechanism for tissue damage is *type III* hypersensitivity: immune complexes of autoantigen and autoantibody deposited from the circulation can cause disease in many sites, such as the skin and vascular system and especially the kidneys. For example, glomerular damage is a feature of systemic lupus erythematosus (SLE) in which autoantibodies to DNA are prominent. By contrast, in Goodpasture's syndrome, kidney damage is caused by antibodies to basement membrane, a *type II* response (see p. 65).

Aetiology of autoimmune diseases

Although the aetiology of autoimmune diseases is unknown, there are some clues as to the 'predisposing factors'. For example, in certain spontaneous animal models of autoimmune thyroiditis and SLE, the animals are genetically programmed to develop autoimmunity, and there is a higher 'risk factor' associated with certain HLA class I and II alleles in man (p. 83). Data from animal models have also suggested that invading microorganisms may be involved in the early stages of disease and that T cells are often involved in both the aetiology and pathogenic processes. In fact, the aetiology is likely to be multifactorial.

As previously discussed, self-tolerance is maintained by a variety of mechanisms (you should now re-read p. 21: Self versus non-self discrimination). A breakdown in any of these mechanisms may lead to autoimmunity. Some potential mechanisms for the breakdown in self-tolerance are shown in Figure 2.

Treatment

Most therapy is directed to alleviating chronic inflammation. Anti-inflammatory drugs are commonly used (e.g. corticosteroids). Removal of antibodies by plasmapheresis has been successful in treating several organ-specific diseases. Immunosuppressive drugs are used to treat both organ and non-organ specific diseases and are described in more detail in the Clinical section and on page 87.

Organ specific diseases		Non-organ specific diseases	
Disease	**Antigen(s)**	**Disease**	**Antigen(s)**
Hashimoto's thyroiditis	Thyroid peroxidase, thyroglobulin	Systemic lupus erythematosus (SLE)	DNA, nuclear antigens
Pernicious anaemia	Intrinsic factor	Chronic active hepatitis	Nuclei, DNA
Insulin-dependent diabetes mellitus	β Cells in pancreas	Scleroderma	Nuclei, lungs, kidney
Addison's disease	Adrenal cells	Primary biliary cirrhosis	Mitochondria
Autoimmune haemolytic anaemia	RBC membrane antigens	Rheumatoid arthritis	IgG (rheumatoid factor), connective tissues
Graves' disease	TSH receptor		
Myasthenia gravis	Acetylcholine receptor	Ankylosing spondylitis	Vertebral
Pemphigus	Intercellular matrix	Multiple sclerosis	Brain and white matter
Guillain–Barré syndrome	Peripheral nerves	Sjögren's syndrome	Exocrine glands, kidney, liver, thyroid
Polymyositis	Muscle		
Several organs affected			
Goodpasture's syndrome	Basement membrane of kidney and lung		
Polyendocrine	Multiple endocrine organ		

Fig. 1 Autoimmune diseases. Although autoimmune diseases are classified as organ or non-organ specific, there is a great deal of overlap between them. For example, diseases such as Goodpasture's syndrome are classified as organ-specific but affect both kidneys and lungs; polyendocrine diseases affect many of the endocrine glands. Note that in many of the non-organ specific diseases the immune response is directed to intracellular antigens and in particular DNA and other nuclear antigens.

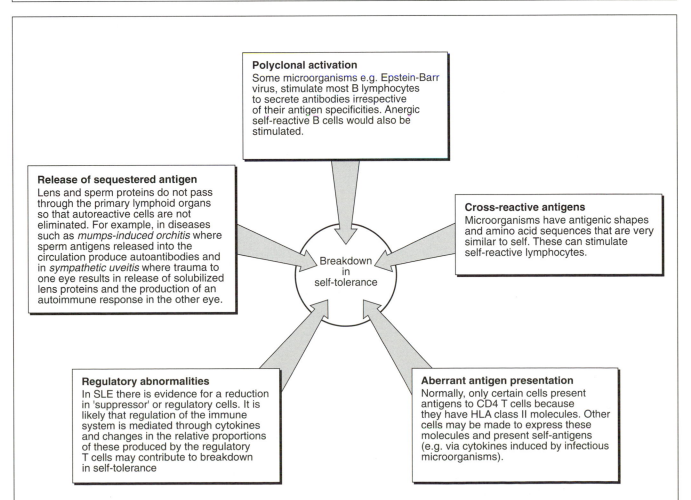

Fig. 2 Possible mechanisms for the breakdown in self-tolerance. A number of mechanisms for breakdown of tolerance have been postulated. All may involve microorganisms.

Infectious Disease

Not all infections cause disease

It is important to separate the concept of *infection* from that of *disease*. In an earlier section (p. 39) we emphasized that the objective of the parasite is to survive and be transmitted. Sometimes this may involve causing pathology; for example, the diarrhoea that helps intestinal parasites to get into water, soil, etc. and infect another host. Coughs and sneezes also spread diseases! Many toxins are used to invade tissues or knock out host defences. Some viruses are obliged to destroy cells in order to spread. And so on. But plenty of microorganisms inhabit the body without causing symptoms, and these could perhaps be regarded as the most successful parasites of all. EB virus in the throat and the normal bacteria of the gut are examples of this.

Disease can be caused at three levels

Look back at page 1 to remind yourself of the three types of host defence:

- external defences, which stop the parasite getting into the body
- natural immune mechanisms, which attempt to eliminate it rapidly
- adaptive immune responses, which back up the natural mechanisms when these fail.

We can identify three corresponding sources of disease (=symptoms = pathology = tissue damage):

- Direct: the simple presence of the parasite in the body may damage tissue.
- Inappropriate or over-active natural immune mechanisms can cause tissue damage.
- Inappropriate or over-active adaptive immune responses can cause tissue damage.

This three-level scheme is illustrated in Figure 1. Some comments on important aspects follow.

Direct tissue damage

Here the main culprits are **cytopathic viruses** and bacterial **exotoxins**. Cytopathic viruses include polio (neurones), rhinoviruses (nasal and pharyngeal mucosa), rotavirus (intestinal epithelium), HIV (T cells). Some bacteria also damage tissue, e.g. *Strep. mutans* (teeth). Malaria parasites are cytopathic for red blood cells. Secretion of exotoxins is a feature of many bacterial infections, the most important being diphtheria, tetanus, staphylococci, streptococci, cholera, *E. coli*, gas gangrene, botulism. The intestinal protozoon *Entamoeba histolytica* also secretes a toxin to help it penetrate the gut wall and there are fungal toxins too.

Damage due to natural immunity

The most dramatic example of this is the widespread effect of **endotoxins**, of which lipopolysaccharide (LPS) from Gram-negative bacteria is the most important. Unlike exotoxins, LPS is a cell wall component, released when the bacteria die. Once released, it stimulates an extraordinary range of immune mechanisms, sometimes with disastrous results (Fig. 2). Very low levels of LPS may, however, be useful in keeping the immune system 'ticking over'. Endotoxins are complex molecules with a highly conserved lipid A portion, a more variable core oligosaccharide and a very polymorphic polysaccharide chain (the bacterial O antigen). The lipid A is the toxic part and many of its effects are due to the induction of cytokines, especially TNF from macrophages. A few micrograms of LPS can be fatal in man, compared to sub-nanogram amounts of botulinum toxin.

Damage due to adaptive immunity (see also p. 45)

The ways in which antibody and T cell responses can lead to disease were usefully classified by Gell and Coombs in 1958, and this scheme is still widely used (Fig. 3). They identified four main types of potentially tissue-damaging response, and immunologists often refer to these simply as type I, type III, etc. They are collectively known as hypersensitivity reactions, and the term immunopathology is also used, although this really applies to the LPS type of response too.

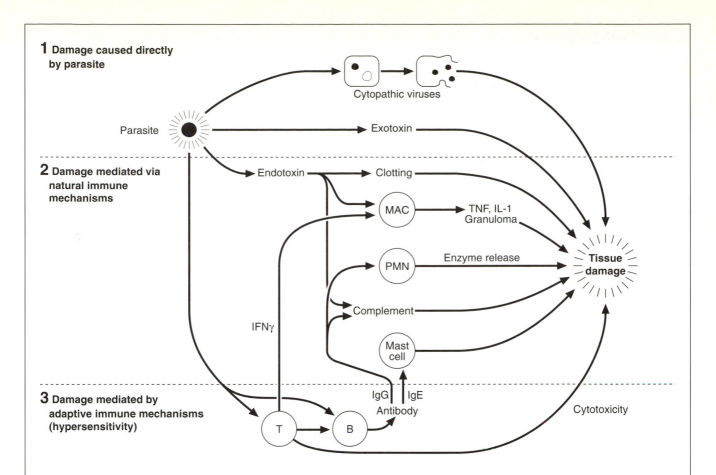

Fig. 1 **Tissue damage during infection can be caused in several different ways.** Note that, just as with the disposal of parasites, natural immune mechanisms are responsible for much of the damage even when lymphocytes are involved. MAC, macrophage; TNF, IL-1, IFNγ, see page 33. See also page 45 for further details.

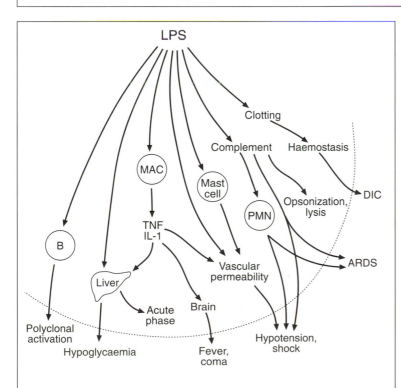

Fig. 2 **Endotoxins activate a wide range of systems with both beneficial and harmful consequences.** In this scheme, the pathological effects are shown outside the dotted line. DIC, disseminated intravascular coagulation, in which multiple thromboses can cause depletion of clotting factors and haemorrhage; ARDS, adult respiratory distress syndrome (a life-threatening complication of severe trauma or infection).

Gell and Coombs type	Examples from infectious disease
I Allergic: IgE + mast cells	Some viral rashes Worms, e.g. ruptured hydatid cyst
II Cytotoxic antibody	Virus-infected cells Autoantibodies streptococci mycoplasma
III Immune complexes	Glomerulonephritis streptococci hepatitis B malaria Allergic alveolitis (Farmer's lung)
IV T cell mediated	Some viral rashes Granuloma TB, leprosy schistosome egg

Fig. 3 **Hypersensitivity of all types may be caused by infection.** See Hypersensitivity, p. 45, for details of mechanisms.
Note! There are also many non-infectious causes of hypersensitivity.

Transplant Rejection

Grafts of skin from one site of the body to another (**autografts**) vascularize and are accepted at the new site. However, skin, cells (e.g. blood) or solid organs (e.g. kidney) transplanted from one person to another (**allografts**) are usually rejected. This is because the adaptive immune system recognizes them as being foreign, just like any microbe.

Transplantation antigens

The antigens on the transplanted cells recognized by the immune system are called **transplantation antigens**. Historically, the strongest of these were called the major histocompatibility complex (MHC) molecules because they determined whether or not tissues were compatible between individuals. We now know that MHC molecules are critical in the recognition of antigens by T cells (see pp. 19 & 31). Why then do these MHC molecules behave as transplantation antigens? The answer is that the MHC molecules differ from person to person.

- Graft rejection. The genetic locus coding for the MHC molecules shows tremendous polymorphism, which means that in the population as a whole, many different allelic forms can occur at this locus. In man, the MHC locus is called the **human leukocyte antigen (HLA) locus** and is made up of four separate subregions, A, B, C and D (Fig. 1). These code for MHC class I (A,B and C) and MHC class II (D) molecules. At each subregion locus, an individual can either be homozygous or heterozygous and since the genes, inherited by simple Mendelian inheritance, are co-dominant, both allelic forms are expressed on the cell surface simultaneously. Each individual can therefore express twelve different combinations if heterozygous at each subregion. Thus, taking all four subregions together, there are more than a million different possible combinations. In fact, the D locus is even more complex and contains further variation (p. 83).
- Transplantation antigens, like microbial antigens, induce an adaptive immune response (with specificity and memory). When graft recipients have rejected tissues/organs once ('first set' rejection), they mount a faster immune response to tissue/organ grafts from the same donor, resulting in an accelerated 'second set' rejection. Tissues/organs obtained from different places in the body stimulate different components of the adaptive immune responses to a variable extent. For example, skin is mainly rejected by cell-mediated responses, whilst blood is mainly removed by antibodies (blood group antibodies). Organ grafts such as kidney are rejected by both anti-HLA antibodies and cell-mediated mechanisms (Fig. 2).

Preventing graft rejection

The severity of graft rejection is mainly determined by the number of genetic differences in the MHC molecules between the donor and recipient. Therefore, the best way to prevent rejection is to select donors and recipients as closely *matched* for the different MHC alleles as possible.

- **Transplantation within families.** Grafts between genetically identical twins are completely accepted, since there are no MHC differences. However, even though not many individuals have an identical twin, a good 'match' is more likely within a family (Fig. 3).
- **Tissue typing.** HLA antigens can be typed by a combination of serological techniques, mainly using B lymphocytes. It is more important to match HLA class II than class I antigens.
- **Immunosuppression.** Except with a perfect match (e.g. identical twins), some immune response will always occur and will need to be suppressed. Drugs which act on lymphocytes and inflammatory processes have largely been replaced by cyclosporin A which acts mainly to inhibit cytokine production (p. 87). Note that these drugs are non-antigen specific, and carry a danger of general immunodeficiency, leading to infection (see p. 53). Antigen-specific approaches (e.g. **tolerance**, p. 21) are showing promise in animal models.

Graft-versus-host (GVH) disease

When the graft contains HLA-incompatible T lymphocytes (e.g. a bone marrow graft), these can attack host tissues, leading to life-threatening **GVH disease**. This can be prevented by removing the T lymphocytes from the marrow and treating the patient with immunosuppressive drugs.

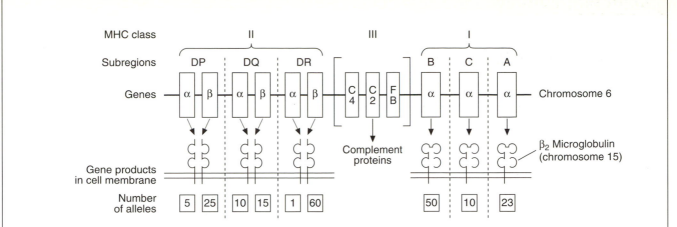

Fig. 1 The human histocompatibility (HLA) locus and its products. Class I and II human leucocyte antigens (HLA) are coded by a gene complex on chromosome 6. It is estimated that there are 400 genes within the whole MHC complex encoding HLA class I, II and III molecules. The non-polymorphic β chain (β$_2$ microglobulin) of the class I molecules is coded for by a gene on chromosome 15. Class III genes code for the complement components C2, C4 and factor B. The number of different alleles for the class I and II molecules is enormous and their gene products are the major histocompatibility antigens recognized as transplantation antigens, whose possible combinations run into millions.

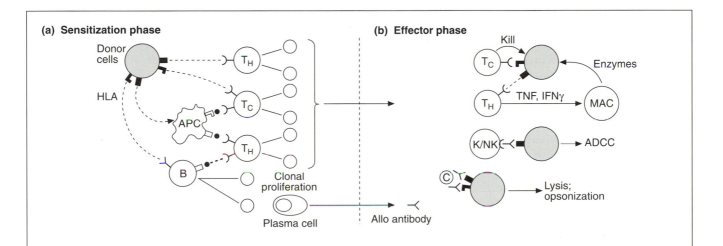

Fig. 2 Graft rejection mechanisms. Rejection can be divided into a **sensitization** and an **effector** phase. (a) Sensitization phase: T$_H$ and T$_C$ are stimulated by coming into contact with foreign class I and II HLA, which are recognized either directly (the T cells recognizing the allografted MHC molecules as self HLA molecules with the polymorphic component acting like a foreign peptide), or indirectly through presentation of the molecules after being processed by host APC or B cells. B cells will also make antibodies (alloantibodies) against graft HLA antigens. Organ grafts frequently contain HLA-bearing *passenger* leucocytes which can be responsible for sensitization. Effector phase: (b). Cell-mediated graft destruction is due to infiltration of the graft with T cells and macrophages. T cells may be directly cytotoxic and cytokines released by T cells (IFNγ, TNF) activate macrophages to release degradative enzymes and enhance expression of HLA on target donor cells, e.g. endothelial vessels of blood vessels. Antibody:complement (C)-mediated, antibody-dependent lysis and opsonization of the grafted cells; antibody-dependent cellular cytotoxicity (ADCC). Minor histocompatibility antigens, not coded for by the HLA locus may also be the targets of the rejection process.

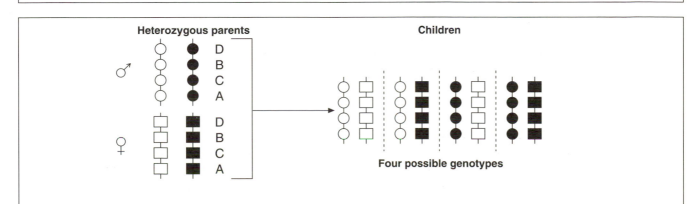

Fig. 3 Inheritance of HLA genes. Since HLA genes lie close together on chromosome 6, they are generally inherited en bloc. In grafts from parents to their offspring or vice versa, at least 50% of the major transplantation antigens will be identical. In sibling to sibling grafts, there is a 1/4 chance that the major transplantation antigens will be identical.

52

Immunodeficiency

Our immune system normally protects us against the diverse array of microorganisms in our environment and defects in the various components of the immune system can lead to life-threatening infections. We become **immunocompromised** as the result of having **immunodeficiency** (ID). The type of infection seen can often give a clue as to what components are defective. For example, extracellular bacterial infections would suggest an antibody defect whilst viral, fungal and intracellular bacterial infections would implicate the T cell system. Infections can be by normal pathogens or, more seriously, by **opportunistic microorganisms** (p. 77). Infections in the immunocompromised are commonly respiratory or gastrointestinal.

Classification of immunodeficiencies

Immunodeficiencies are classified as either **primary** or **secondary**. Primary ID is the result of an inherent **congenital** defect in the components of the immune system or their products. Secondary ID results from the effects of external agents or breakdown in other body systems which affect the immune system and is sometimes referred to as **acquired**.

Primary (or congenital) immunodeficiency

This is rare, but can result from defects in either natural or adaptive immunity. Deficiencies can occur at various levels, from stem cells to more differentiated precursors resulting in **neutropenias** or, for lymphocytes, **severe combined immune deficiencies** (SCID: Fig. 1). Deficiencies in neutrophil function can also occur, ranging from defective chemotaxis to failure of intracellular bacterial killing (Fig. 2). Various complement components can also be deficient (Fig. 3). Isolated antibody and cell-mediated deficiencies occur when B and T cells fail to develop or function normally. B cells can be 'arrested' at different stages of normal B cell development. (e.g. **Bruton's disease**, where no B cells are produced, Fig. 4). In **Di George syndrome**, the thymus fails to develop, resulting in an absence of T cells. T cells may also be affected in the thymus by deficiency in enzymes involved in the DNA salvage pathway (Fig. 5).

Secondary (or acquired) immunodeficiency

These are by far the most common. Predisposing factors leading to secondary ID include:

- **Malnutrition**: protein-calorie malnutrition and lack of certain dietary elements (e.g. iron, zinc) is world-wide the most serious predisposing factor for secondary ID.
- **Loss** of cellular/humoral components: e.g. lymphocytes lost in the intestine in intestinal lymphangiectasia; antibodies, lost into the urine in nephrotic syndrome.
- **Tumours**: the direct effect of tumours of the immune system itself or other cells.
- **Cytotoxic drugs/irradiation**: these are widely used for inhibiting tumour cell growth but simultaneously damage immune cells, e.g. stem cells and rapidly dividing lymphocytes in the primary lymphoid organs. Prior to AIDS, cytotoxic drug treatments and tumours were the most important predisposing factors leading to secondary ID in the western world.
- **Other diseases** such as diabetes are associated with infections.
- **Infections** such as malaria inhibit immune responses. Human immunodeficiency viruses (HIV) cause a particularly severe form of immunodeficiency (AIDS: p. 81).

Treatment of immunodeficiency

Antibiotic therapy is the standard treatment for infections. Passive gammaglobulin therapy is also used for antibody deficiencies. Bone marrow transplantation has been successfully used for reconstitution of normal phagocytic function in chronic granulomatous disease (CGD) and of B and T cells in SCID. Fetal liver and thymus grafts have also been successfully used. The ultimate treatment, at least for primary ID, will be gene replacement therapy where the identified faulty gene will be replaced in the patient's stem cells with a 'normal' gene; this has already been tried for ADA deficiency and (in mice) for cystic fibrosis.

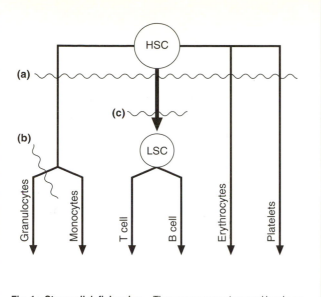

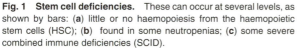

Fig. 1 Stem cell deficiencies. These can occur at several levels, as shown by bars: (**a**) little or no haemopoiesis from the haemopoietic stem cells (HSC); (**b**) found in some neutropenias; (**c**) some severe combined immune deficiencies (SCID).

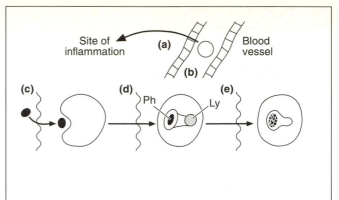

Fig. 2 Defects in normal phagocytic function. (**a**) Neutrophils are unable to respond to chemotactic stimuli, e.g. from complement-mediated opsonization (lazy leucocyte syndrome). (**b**) Neutrophils are unable to marginate because they lack specific adhesion molecules to bind to the blood vessel endothelium (leucocyte adhesion deficiency, LAD). (**c**) Bacteria are not opsonized (e.g. in the classical complement pathway mediated through C1; see C deficiency). (**d**) Phagosomes (Ph) containing phagocytosed microbes do not fuse with lysosomes (Ly) containing killing agents (Chediak–Higashi syndrome). (**e**) Lysosomes do not contain important cytotoxic agents for intracellular killing. For example, oxygen free radicals in chronic granulomatous disease (CGD); myeloperoxidase deficiency.

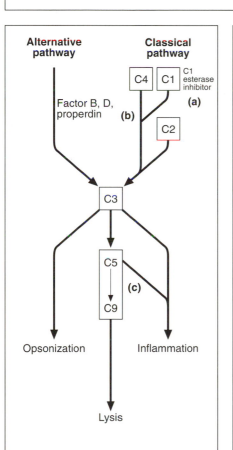

Fig. 3 Deficiencies in complement components. Deficiencies are generally classified into three major kinds. (a) C1 esterase inhibitor deficiency, the commonest inherited complement deficiency, results in hereditary angiodema; (b) deficiencies in the early components which can lead to opsonin defects; (**c**) deficiencies in the late components (membrane attack complex), commonly accompanied by neisserrial infections.

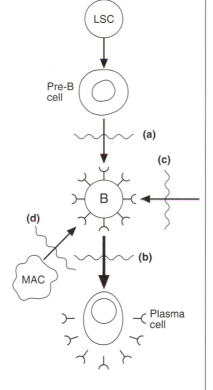

Fig. 4 B cell (antibody) deficiencies. (**a**) Pre-B cells containing cytoplasmic IgM fail to develop into mature B cells expressing surface antibody receptors (Bruton's disease). This results in no B cells in the circulation and no antibodies (agammaglobulinaemia). Other defects are the result of the inability of the mature B cells to develop into plasma cells. This may be the result of (**b**) inherent B cell deficiencies; (**c**) lack of T cell help; (**d**) accessory cell function defects. Selective deficiencies in specific classes/subclasses also occur. The most common immunodeficiency is selective IgA deficiency and is present (usually asymptomatically) in 1/600 individuals!

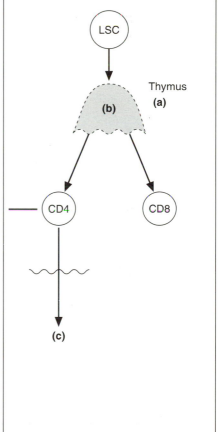

Fig. 5 T cell deficiencies. These occur due to: (**a**) No thymus (thymic aplasia, Di George syndrome) due to lack of development from the 3rd and 4th pharyngeal pouches; also affects para-thyroids and some blood vessels. (**b**) Accumulation of adenosine or guanosine due to defective adenosine deaminase (ADA) or purine nucleoside phosphorylase (PNP) respectively (also results in SCID). (**c**) Defective production of IFNγ has been reported.

Tutorial 4

This short immunopathology section should have made you aware of the close links between microbiology, immunology and histopathology (morbid anatomy), none of which can be studied in total isolation. Test your knowledge with the following questions (answers opposite).

Questions

1. What elements do the response to infection and the response to injury have in common?

2. What can happen if antigen is injected into the skin of an immune patient?

3. What is the significance of finding an autoantibody in a patient's blood?

4. Distinguish between exotoxins and endotoxins.

5. What advantage is there for an infectious organism in making its host ill?

6. How do we know that rejection of a kidney graft is an adaptive immune response?

7. Distinguish between primary and secondary immunodeficiency.

8. What immune defects might predispose a patient to bacterial infection?

Further reading

Most of the topics covered in this section will also be dealt with in textbooks of pathology, though sometimes without the emphasis on the role of the immune system. The following are particularly worth reading.

Woolf N 1986 Cell, tissue and disease, 2nd edn. Bailliere Tindall, London, 503 pp. A very clearly written textbook of basic pathology, excellent on the areas where pathology and immunology overlap. A book to buy.

Austin Gresham G 1971 A colour atlas of general pathology. Wolfe Publishing, London, 365 pp. The Wolfe colour atlases are an excellent source of vivid pictures. This one illustrates inflammation, though not from the immunological angle.

Holgate S T, Church M K (eds) 1993 Allergy. Gower Medical, London. All you could possibly want to know about type I hypersensitivity, from over 30 authors, with hundreds of colour pictures and a slide-atlas.

Glynn L E, Holborow E J 1965 Autoimmunity and disease. Blackwell Scientific, Oxford, 420 pp. A classic text, quite out-of-date in many respects, but showing the way the phenomenon of autoimmunity was used to make deductions about normal immunity — including a foreshadowing of the distinction between T and B cells which 'officially' occurred a year later.

Humphrey J H, White R G 1965 Immunology for students of medicine, 2nd edn. Blackwell Scientific, Oxford, 450 pp. Another classic, the first real textbook of immunology, with many interesting and scholarly discussions of immunopathology, still unbeaten for its 'historical' flavour.

Gell P G H, Coombs R R A 1963 Clinical aspects of immunology, 2nd edn. Blackwell Scientific, Oxford, 1356 pp. The second edition of this classic book (now in its fifth edition) is famous for the first appearance of the Gell and Coombs classification of hypersensitivities.

Answers

1. Degranulation of mast cells, activation of complement, release of prostaglandins and leukotrienes, all leading to increased vascular permeability; influx of fluid and cells, especially PMN; later influx of macrophages and progression to either healing or chronic inflammation, depending on whether the initial stimulus has persisted or not. In particular situations, one or other of the above may predominate.

2. It depends on the patient's immune status. High levels of specific IgE on mast cells will lead to mast cell degranulation, with a local 'wheal and flare' response in minutes (type I or immediate hypersensitivity); IgG in the tissues may lead to local necrosis (type III or Arthus reaction); T cell immunity may cause delayed (type IV) responses of various kinds, typically a red swelling 2–3 days later.

3. It may be the cause of the patient's disease (e.g. anti-acetylcholine receptor in myasthenia gravis, anti-TSH receptor in Graves' disease); it may be a sign that a particular organ or subcellular component is affected (e.g. anti-adrenal in Addison's disease, anti-mitochondria in primary biliary cirrhosis); or it may be a pointer to a particular infection (e.g. cardiolipin antibodies in syphilis).

4. Exotoxins are proteins secreted by certain microbes (mostly bacteria but also some fungi and protozoa) which may help them to spread or to evade defence mechanisms. Examples: tetanus, diphtheria, botulism. Endotoxins are integral constituents of the cell wall of Gram-negative bacteria, usually lipopolysaccharides, which may be released when the bacteria die and then stimulate numerous activities, e.g. clotting, complement activation, TNF release from macrophages and, in extreme cases, shock. Weight for weight, exotoxins are up to a million times more lethal than endotoxins. Exotoxins make excellent vaccines, endotoxins do not.

5. Sometimes the symptoms of infection may be directly beneficial to the invading microbe. For example, tissue damage may be induced by the organism in the process of spreading through the tissues (e.g. streptococcal hyaluronidase), spreading from one cell to another (e.g. cytopathic viruses) or spreading to another host (e.g. organisms that induce coughing, sneezing, or diarrhoea). But remember that many symptoms are caused by the immune system (immunopathology), while many infectious organisms do not cause disease at all (e.g. the normal gut flora).

6. Rejection of a kidney (or skin, etc.) graft shows the classic features of adaptive immunity: memory and specificity. Thus a second graft carrying the same HLA antigens will be rejected faster than the first one, but a second graft with different HLA antigens will be rejected on the normal 'first set' time-scale, starting about a week after grafting. This delay is another sign that adaptive, rather than natural, immunity is at work. Further proof comes from the fact that animals or humans without lymphocytes cannot reject grafts, however foreign.

7. A patient is born with primary immunodeficiency, but acquires secondary immunodeficiency. Thus 'primary' implies a genetic defect (which may or may not be inherited), whereas 'secondary' implies an external cause, such as drugs, other diseases, etc.

8. Extracellular bacteria: antibody deficiency, complement deficiency, defects in phagocytes, especially PMN. Intracellular bacteria: T cell defects.

56

Immunology in Medicine

It may seem at first sight that most doctors can get along quite well without knowing much immunology. But, in fact, any doctor, whether house surgeon, psychiatrist or general practitioner, may be confronted at any time by a patient whose problem can only be understood and correctly managed if immunological principles are borne in mind — along with everything else!

Four reasons for thinking immunologically

Practically any presentation may be the sign of a disease which:

- Results from some **deficiency** in the immune system. This may range from an annoying series of skin infections to life-threatening pneumonia, and there is little chance that treatment will be effective unless the immunodeficiency is properly investigated. It is, of course, equally important to establish that a particular symptom is *not* due to an immunological defect.
- Results from **over-activity** of some part of the immune system. Here the range is vast: from mild hay-fever to progressively fatal kidney failure or arthritis. Or there may be vague debilitating symptoms of no obvious cause. Are they psychiatric or immunological? Only someone with an understanding of both disciplines is likely to be able to decide.
- Benefits from immunological laboratory tests in arriving at the **diagnosis** even though not primarily immunological. Chronic liver disease is an excellent example. Medical textbooks list ten or more causes of chronic hepatitis, some of which are primarily due to infection, drugs or inherited conditions but which trigger off characteristic immunological changes; to make a diagnosis in such a case without sending a serum sample to the immunology laboratory would be very unwise. The same applies to anaemia, arthritis, diabetes, nephritis, skin diseases, etc. etc. The immune system responds to almost any deviation from normal health and may be the first pointer to the cause of the trouble.
- Requires treatment by **vaccination** or a **transplant**, neither of which could possibly be contemplated without an understanding of immunological principles.

Further reading

Clinical immunology is of course a much larger subject than the following few pages can cover, and anyone who wishes to specialize in this or the related fields of infectious disease, transplantation, microbiology, haematology, etc. should possess at least one of the textbooks listed below.

Chapel H, Heaney M 1993 Essentials of clinical immunology, 3rd edn. Blackwell Scientific, Oxford, 336 pp. An excellent system-based guide to the subject, very clearly written and illustrated, with case reports and self-tests conveying a vivid feel for the activities of the clinical and laboratory immunologist.

Brostoff J, Scadding G, Male D, Roitt I (eds) 1991 Clinical immunology. Gower Medical, London. Thirty chapters by 39 authors, with hundreds of striking colour illustrations, which are also available as a useful slide atlas. Complements the popular basic volume Immunology from the same publishers.

Stites D, Terr A, Parslow T G (eds) 1994 Basic and clinical immunology, 8th edn. Prentice-Hall, London, 870pp. A multi-author American book, lively and up-to-date, with sections on laboratory tests and therapy, very good value.

Lachmann P, Peters K, Rosen F, Walport M (eds) 1993 Clinical aspects of immunology, 5th edn. Blackwell Scientific, Oxford, 2176 pp. A three-volume multi-author compendium of immunology, including basic and technical chapters, written in the form of definitive expert review articles with substantial reference sections. Not extensively illustrated. This represents the 'scholarly' end of the range.

Immunology for the clinician: a summary

In the following pages, the immunological aspects of medicine are considered by organ/system, as they are usually encountered in the teaching course. Below, we summarize the most important conditions along immunological lines, to bring out the different ways in which the immunologist can be involved (for an explanation of the abbreviations, see the relevant pages).

Immunodeficiency diseases (refresh your memory by re-reading p. 53)

Remember that primary immunodeficiency is rare, that in about half the children affected no defect is ever found and that, when it is, it is more often in the phagocytic cells. Primary deficiency of antibody is very rare and that of T cells even more so. The respiratory system is overwhelmingly the commonest site of infection. Treatment is difficult, except in the case of hypogammaglobulinaemia (passive Ig).

Immunodeficiency in adults is almost always secondary to some other condition (drugs, infection, lymphoproliferative disease, etc.). Quite often infection is with normally harmless opportunists, such as pseudomonas, pneumocystis, CMV or yeasts.

Hypersensitivity diseases (re-read p. 45)

Type I   Allergic asthma, anaphylaxis, drug allergy, food allergy? eczema?
Type II   Autoantibodies in Graves' disease, myasthenia gravis, haemolytic anaemia, thrombocytopenia, pemphigus, Goodpasture's syndrome, adrenalitis?
Note! Finding an autoantibody does *not* mean it is the cause of the disease.
Type III   Immune complexes in kidney, skin, blood vessels, eye, serum sickness
Type IV   T cell immunity in chronic infections, contact dermatitis and perhaps in sarcoidosis, scleroderma, psoriasis, coeliac disease, Crohn's disease, ulcerative colitis, Hashimoto's thyroiditis, eczema, type 1 diabetes.
Note! It is often difficult to disentangle type III and IV, e.g. in farmer's lung.

Diagnostic value of autoantibodies

- Connective tissue diseases: rheumatoid (anti Ig); SLE (anti-dsDNA); Sjögren's (La, Ro)
- Skin: scleroderma (ANA); bullous diseases (Ig in biopsy section)
- Liver: chronic active hepatitis (DNA, smooth muscle); primary biliary cirrhosis (mitochondrial)
- Blood: pernicious anaemia (IF); haemolytic anaemia (antiglobulin test)
- Pancreas: type I diabetes (islet cells).

Vaccination

- Standard for: diphtheria, tetanus, pertussis, polio, measles, mumps, rubella
- At risk: hepatitis B, influenza, VZV, typhoid, cholera, BCG, yellow fever, pneumococci, meningococci, haemophilus, rabies (post-exposure).
- Passive antibody for: diphtheria, tetanus, clostridia, snakebite, rabies, VZV.

Transplantation

- Kidney, bone marrow (GVH!) and more rarely heart, liver, pancreas
- Need for HLA matching, immunosuppressive drugs.

HLA-disease links

Only of diagnostic value in ankylosing spondylitis (B27); others of academic interest (e.g. B8/DR3 in autoimmunity).

Respiratory Disease

Being literally open to the outside air, the respiratory tract is exposed to vast numbers of inhaled microorganisms, but the lung itself is normally sterile thanks to a combination of three major protective mechanisms: the 'mucociliary escalator', alveolar macrophages and antibody (especially IgA). If these are defective, severe repeated lung infections can result.

Upper respiratory tract infections

Colds are caused by a variety of viruses; the rapid recovery is probably mainly due to interferon and the lack of immunity to extensive serotypic variation. Sore throats are also mainly viral, but there are some important bacterial causes too (Fig. 1). Both types of organism can spread to sinuses, middle ear and lower respiratory tract. Immunity is depressingly ineffective.

Pneumonia and tuberculosis

The classic causative organism is *Strep. pneumoniae*, but a variety of other bacteria and viruses can cause pneumonia (Fig. 2). Roughly half of patients with repeated bacterial pneumonia have some form of **immunodeficiency**, predominantly affecting antibody (Fig. 3). Conversely, respiratory infections are by far the commonest complication of antibody deficiency. In tuberculosis, on the other hand, defects involving T cells have the most serious effects — the current exacerbation of TB in areas affected by AIDS being an example. However over-reaction of T cells is also harmful through the induction of granulomas (an example of type IV hypersensitivity, see p. 45). Strangely enough, despite over a century of research, the exact mechanism of successful anti-TB immunity is not understood, although it clearly involves T cells and macrophages. Note that vaccines exist for *S. pneumoniae* and tuberculosis but their use is restricted to those most at risk (see p. 79).

Sarcoidosis and other systemic diseases

This mysterious disease presents with non-necrotic granulomas in the lung and other organs, the principal immunological finding being macrophage activation combined with a deficiency of T cell functions. No microorganism has been identified but, as in some of the skin diseases (see p. 69), an infectious agent of some kind is suspected. The lung is frequently involved in other systemic granulomatous and vasculitic diseases, e.g. Wegener's granulomatosis and SLE, and a wide range of other chronic conditions can lead ultimately to pulmonary fibrosis (Fig. 4).

Hypersensitivity and asthma

Like the kidney, the lung is very susceptible to immunopathological reactions; some examples are listed in Figure 5. Note, however, that it is not always easy to place these precisely in the Gell and Coombs' classification. For instance, **extrinsic allergic alveolitis** (Fig. 6), of which 'farmer's lung' is typical, shows features of both immune complex-mediated (type III) and cell-mediated (type IV) hypersensitivity. At least 50% of **asthma** is due to type I (allergic) hypersensitivity, and the allergen can often be identified by an immediate skin test or by bronchial challenge (under medical supervision!). These patients have raised IgE and eosinophil levels in the blood, a common finding in allergy. However in the other 50% of patients these are not found, skin tests are negative and the cause is not precisely known; this is known as intrinsic asthma (Fig. 7).

Acute respiratory failure and ARDS

Acute respiratory failure can be of pulmonary, cardiac or neurological origin, but one form has immunological implications; this is the **adult respiratory distress syndrome** that can occur during infection or following severe trauma or surgery. Even with the best intensive care, up to 50% of ARDS patients die. Neutrophils, macrophages, complement and cytokines (e.g. TNF) all seem to be involved in the acute generalized pulmonary oedema, which may represent a common response of the lung to a wide variety of insults (Fig. 8).

Common cold
Rhinovirus
Coronavirus
Echovirus
Coxsackie virus

Pharyngitis
Cold viruses
Adenovirus
EB virus
Influenza,* para-influenza
Strep. pyogenes (GpA)
N. gonorrhoeae
*C. diphtheria**
*Haemophilus influenzae**

Fig. 1 Many viruses and some bacteria cause infections of the upper respiratory tract. * Vaccine available.

Viruses
Influenza, para-influenza
Respiratory syncitial virus
Measles
Cytomegalovirus
Adeno-, rhinoviruses
Varicella
Mycoplasma
Chlamydia trachomatis

Bacteria
Strep. pneumoniae
H. influenzae
*Staph. aureus**
Legionella pneumophilia
M. tuberculosis
*Klebsiella pneumoniae**
*Pseudomonas**
*Enterobacteria**

Fig. 2 The major causes of pneumonia. * These organisms are particularly likely to cause pneumonia in hospitalized patients.

Antibody deficiencies
Bacterial pneumonias (see Fig. 2)
Pseudomonas *
Klebsiella *

Phagocyte defects
Bacterial and fungal infections
Aspergillus *
Cryptococcus

T cell deficiencies
Viral pneumonias
Tuberculosis
Fungi:　*Candida* *
　　　　Pneumocystis *

Malnutrition
Tuberculosis
Pneumocystis *
Strongyloides *

Fig. 3 Respiratory infection is the commonest complication of immuno-deficiency. The pattern of infection depends on the type of defect. *Some organisms are only pathogenic in immunodeficient patients; these are known as 'opportunists' and are often difficult to treat.

Granulomatous
Sarcoidosis
Tuberculosis
Extrinsic allergic alveolitis
Inhalation
　Silica
　Asbestos
　Beryllium

Systemic vasculitis
SLE
Wegener's granulomatosis
Rheumatoid arthritis
Polyarteritis

Post-pneumonia
Irradiation
Cryptogenic (i.e. idiopathic)

Fig. 4 Many conditions can give rise to lung fibrosis. As in most forms of chronic inflammation, macrophages and fibroblasts are the predominant cells involved.

Type I (allergic)
Hay fever
Allergic asthma
Tropical eosinophilia

Type II (cytotoxic antibody)
Goodpasture's syndrome

Type III (immune-complex mediated)
Extrinsic allergic alveolitis
Vasculitis (see Fig. 4)

Type IV (T cell mediated)
Granulomatous diseases (see Fig. 4)
Extrinsic allergic alveolitis

Cytokine mediated
ARDS?

Fig. 5 Many respiratory conditions are immunopathological in origin. Examples are shown here of all the major types of mechanism.

Bacteria (actinomycetes)
Farmer's lung
Bagassosis
Mushroom worker's lung

Fungi
Malt worker's lung
Tobacco worker's lung
Maple bark disease
Cheese worker's lung
Thatched roof disease

Animals
Allergy to laboratory rats, mice, etc.
Pigeon breeder's disease
Bird fancier's lung
Furrier's lung

Fig. 6 Extrinsic allergic alveolitis (in the US, 'hypersensitivity pneumonitis'). This can be caused by a variety of inhaled antigens associated with particular occupations. In most cases the antigen responsible has not been precisely identified. IgE is *not* involved.

Extrinsic (allergic: type I)	**Intrinsic** (idiopathic; type II)
Usually childhood onset	Often adult onset
Atopic family history	Viral infection
Positive skin test	Drugs (e.g. aspirin)
Bronchial provocation test	Cold
Seasonal incidence (pollen)	Smoke, fumes
Non-seasonal	Exercise
animals	Stress
house dust mites	
seafood	
drugs (e.g. penicillin)	

Fig. 7 Bronchial asthma or 'reversible airways obstruction'. This is usually classified as allergic or non-allergic (idiopathic) but considerable overlaps occur. Some features of the two types are shown.

Septic shock (especially Gram-negative)
Severe trauma; burns
Near-drowning
Post surgical
Gastric acid aspiration
Drug overdose
Fat embolism (e.g. post-fracture)
CNS injury
Massive transfusion

Fig. 8 Adult respiratory distress syndrome. Universally known as 'ARDS', this is a life-threatening response to numerous acute emergencies. Those cases due to Gram-negative bacteria may be helped by antibodies to endotoxin, but this is controversial.

The Gut and Liver

Like the skin and lungs, the gut is an interface with the outside world — for food as well as infectious organisms (which sometimes arrive simultaneously!); it is quite an achievement to respond immunologically to the latter and not the former. The gut is well furnished with lymphoid tissue (see p. 15 to be reminded about MALT and p. 23 for the special properties of IgA), and several of its major diseases appear to be due to an immunopathological response. For convenience, these are usually considered according to their predominant anatomical location.

Mouth and salivary glands

The dry mouth of **Sjögren's syndrome** (see p. 73) is due to destruction of salivary glands, with infiltration by (mainly) T lymphocytes (Fig. 1*a*). The cause is unknown.

Stomach and jejunum

Type A gastritis (Fig. 1*b*), a major cause of **pernicious anaemia** due to malabsorption of vitamin B_{12}, shows all the signs of being an autoimmune disease (Fig. 2) though the aetiology is unknown. It may occur as part of a polyendocrine syndrome (see p. 63).

Coeliac disease, in which the jejunal mucosa is infiltrated by T lymphocytes and normal villous structure is lost (Fig. 1*c*) leading to malabsorption of fat, vitamins, etc., is the most convincing example of hypersensitivity to a food component — in this case the α-gliadin component of gluten, from wheat flour. T cell responses to a small peptide are suspected, but not proved, to be the cause. There is a strong association with the bullous skin disease, dermatitis herpetiformis (see p. 69).

Ileum and colon

Two chronic inflammatory conditions affecting the lower intestine may represent immune responses to food or infection, though this is not proved. They are **Crohn's disease** (which can also affect other parts of the gut) and **ulcerative colitis** (Figs 1*d* & 1*e*). The characteristic granulomas of Crohn's disease have suggested to some workers a mycobacterial cause. Abnormal expression of MHC class II antigens, found on the diseased mucosa, may result in the presentation of bowel antigens to T cells (a similar mechanism may operate in the thyroid in Graves' disease).

The liver and hepatitis

Elimination of hepatitis B virus is initiated by a cytotoxic T cell response to the infected hepatocytes; there is, therefore, a delicate balance between excessive liver destruction (acute fulminant hepatitis, fortunately rare) and failure to eliminate the virus (chronic infection), with normal recovery poised between these extremes. Chronic infection is the commonest complication (up to 10% of patients and 50% with the recently discovered hepatitis C), and as well as leading to persistent carriage of the virus (which keeps the infection going in the community) it can lead to **chronic active hepatitis (CAH)** which may in turn lead to cirrhosis (see Fig. 3 for a list of other causes of CAH, including the important autoimmune variety). The carrier state is especially common when the infection occurs in young children, as it usually does in the Far East. One unexpected benefit was that the blood of carriers was the source of the first successful hepatitis B **vaccine**, since the non-infectious surface coat is produced in vast excess; the vaccine is now manufactured by recombinant DNA technology (i.e. 'genetically engineered').

The bile ducts

Lymphocytic infiltration of the bile ducts, with granuloma formation, characterizes **primary biliary cirrhosis** (Fig. 1*f*), in which the most striking immunological finding is autoantibodies to mitochondria – probably to an enzyme found in both mitochondria and some bacteria (Fig. 4).

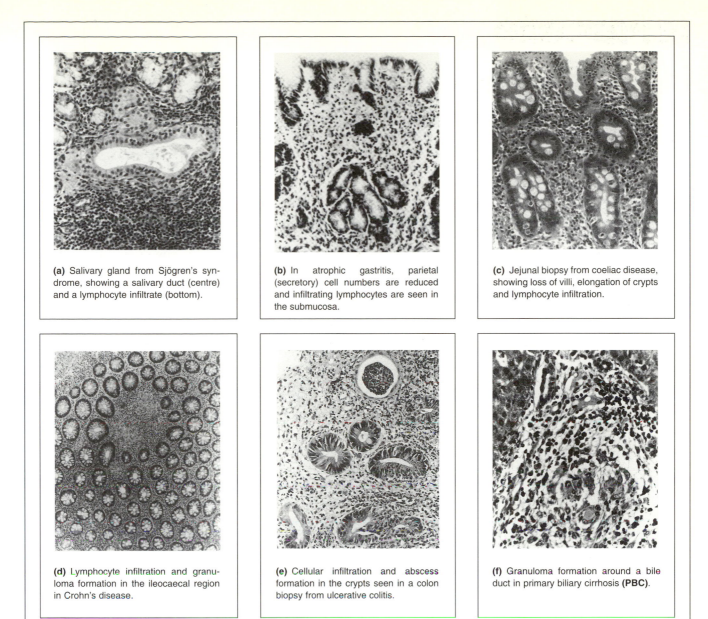

(a) Salivary gland from Sjögren's syndrome, showing a salivary duct (centre) and a lymphocyte infiltrate (bottom).

(b) In atrophic gastritis, parietal (secretory) cell numbers are reduced and infiltrating lymphocytes are seen in the submucosa.

(c) Jejunal biopsy from coeliac disease, showing loss of villi, elongation of crypts and lymphocyte infiltration.

(d) Lymphocyte infiltration and granuloma formation in the ileocaecal region in Crohn's disease.

(e) Cellular infiltration and abscess formation in the crypts seen in a colon biopsy from ulcerative colitis.

(f) Granuloma formation around a bile duct in primary biliary cirrhosis **(PBC)**.

Fig. 1 **Increased numbers of lymphocytes are the hallmark of a variety of diseases affecting the gut and related tissues.** Sometimes granuloma formation follows (Crohn's, PBC) and sometimes destruction predominates — either atrophy of villi (atrophic gastritis, coeliac disease) or abscess formation and necrosis (ulcerative colitis). The pathogenesis is not really understood in any of these.

Type A gastritis (body, not fundus)
Low:
  acid
  intrinsic factor
  B_{12} absorption
Autoantibodies to:
  intrinsic factor (blocking + binding)
  gastric parietal cells
Associated with:
  thyroid autoimmunity
  adrenal, parathyroid autoimmunity
Responds to steroids

Fig. 2 **The failure to absorb vitamin B_{12} in pernicious anaemia is due to depletion of Intrinsic Factor (IF).** This is caused partly by anti-IF antibodies and partly by destruction of gastric parietal cells (probably by T cells).

Autoimmune (female > male)
  Autoantibodies to:
    smooth muscle
    mitochondria
    DNA
    liver antigens
  High serum IgG

Persistent hepatitis B infection
Persistent hepatitis C (20% of cases)
Wilson's disease
Haemochromatosis
Drugs; alcohol (?)
α-₁ antitrypsin deficiency

Fig. 3 **Chronic active hepatitis, defined by lymphocytic infiltration around the portal tracts, can be due to a variety of causes.** Worldwide, persistent infection is the commonest form, but in Europe the autoimmune type predominates. All may progress to cirrhosis.

Primary
  Portal granuloma (CD4, CD8 T cells)
  Autoantibodies to:
    mitochondria
    DNA, liver antigens
  Raised serum IgM associated with:
    Sjögren's (SICCA) syndrome
    systemic sclerosis(CREST syndrome)
    chronic active hepatitis
Secondary to biliary obstruction

Fig. 4 **Biliary cirrhosis can be primary or secondary.** The primary disease, commonest in middle-aged females, appears to be due to autoimmunity, perhaps induced by bacterial infection.

Endocrine Disease

The endocrine organs are remarkably susceptible to **autoimmunity**; indeed autoimmunity is responsible for a considerable proportion of endocrine disease. Though endocrine autoimmunity is usually organ-specific, some patients have symptoms of more than one endocrine disease, and others — especially their relatives — may have one or more autoantibodies without disease suggesting a quite complex genetic basis. Like autoimmunity in general, these diseases are more common in women. Endocrine autoimmunity may be cellular or humoral; in the latter case, the autoantibodies may be against endocrine cells, hormone receptors or the hormones themselves. The most important clinical conditions are described briefly below.

- **Thyroid autoimmunity** was the first to be recognized (in 1957). The most clear-cut syndromes are due to autoantibodies against the thyroid-stimulating hormone (TSH) receptor, which may be (1) **stimulating**, causing hyperthyroidism (thyrotoxicosis/Graves' disease) or simple overgrowth (goitre), either alone or in combination, or (2) **blocking**, causing hypothyroidism (myxoedema). Graves' disease is interesting in being one of the conditions (myasthenia gravis is another) in which transfer of autoantibody from mother to fetus can cause transient symptoms in the newborn; the exophthalmos is suspected of being autoimmune too, but the mechanism is quite unknown. In Hashimoto's thyroiditis, a progressive cellular autoimmune response to thyroid antigens is seen associated with areas of follicle destruction and regeneration and variable effects on thyroid function (usually not affected). For details of the other antibodies found in thyroid conditions, see Figure 1.

- **Diabetes** of the insulin-dependent type (type I) appears to be due to autoimmune destruction of pancreatic β cells, mainly by T cells though various autoantibodies are also found which may be useful in predicting prognosis (see Fig. 2). There is a strong link with MHC antigens 3 and 4 at the DR locus, while DR2 and 5 seem to confer protection (see Fig. 3 and p. 83 for other examples of this 'HLA association'). Many consider that the disease may be initiated by viral infection, and the incidence is on the increase, especially in colder countries. Immunodeficiency is common in diabetic patients resulting in a serious predisposition to bacterial and fungal infection.

- **Adrenal** insufficiency (Addison's disease) is nowadays mainly due to autoimmunity, though previously TB was the commonest cause. Lymphocyte infiltration into the adrenal cortex (sparing the medulla) and an association with HLA DR3 and 4 suggest a similar pathology to type I diabetes, and indeed the two diseases, together with thyroiditis, are often associated. There is some evidence for anti-ACTH receptor autoantibodies, both with blocking (Addison's disease) and stimulating (Cushing's syndrome) actions. See Figure 4 for details of these and other endocrine autoantibodies.

- **Other endocrine organs** can also be affected. Hypopituitarism, hypoparathyroidism, male infertility and premature menopause have all been associated with autoimmunity, though it is probably not a major cause of any of these complaints. Remember that sperm antigens develop well after birth, so that normal tolerance (see p. 21) does not develop. Damage to the testis (trauma, mumps) may release these antigens, giving rise to autoimmune orchitis (Fig. 4 and p. 47).

- **Polyendocrine disease** is the name given to syndromes in which more than two of the above conditions occur together, sometimes also associated with pernicious anaemia due to atrophic gastritis (see p. 61). Certain combinations are commonest (see Fig. 5) and there are links with HLA DR3 and also with fungal infection (*Candida*).

Treatment of endocrine failure

In principle, endocrine failure is easily treatable by simply replacing the hormone. However in diabetes, this does not prevent all the complications (e.g. vasculitis); immunosuppression and pancreatic grafts have both been tried but neither is standard. Thyrotoxicosis is treated by ablating the thyroid either surgically or with radio-iodine, but minor hyperthyroidism responds well to anti-thyroid drugs and beta-blockers. Again, not all the complications are relieved (e.g. exophthalmos can persist).

Antigen	Disease association
TSH receptor	
stimulating	Hyperthyroidism, Goitre
blocking	Hypothyroidism
Eye muscle?	Exophthalmos
Fat cells?	Pretibial myxoedema
Thyroglobulin	Hashimoto's thyroiditis
	Myxoedema
	Thyrotoxicosis
Thyroid peroxidase	Hashimoto's thyroiditis
('microsomal')	Myxoedema
	Thyrotoxicosis

Fig. 1 Thyroid autoimmunity. Many autoantibodies are found in thyroid patients, but most are diagnostic of thyroid disease rather than one particular condition, and all may be secondary to organ damage by cellular mechanisms. Only antibodies against the TSH receptor are firmly established as pathogenic.

Antigen	Disease association
Islet cells	
cytoplasmic	Type I (before onset)
surface	Type I
Insulin receptor	Insulin resistance
Insulin	Type I (before onset)
	Use of foreign insulin
	Insulin resistance

Fig. 2 Various antibodies are found in diabetes and may be valuable in predicting the onset and course of disease. However they are generally considered to be secondary to islet damage and/or insulin release rather than the primary cause of the disease.

Disease	Associated HLA antigen DR	Associated HLA antigen B	Relative risk
Diabetes	3,4	8	5–10
Graves' disease	3	8	2–4
Addison's disease	3	8	6
Ankylosing spondylitis		27	90
Reiter's disease		27	33
Juvenile RA	5	27	3
Coeliac disease	3,7	8	8–11
Goodpasture's syndrome	2		13
Narcolepsy	2		130

Fig. 3 Several endocrine diseases are associated with particular HLA antigens. However, as can be seen from the table, these associations are not as strong as are seen with some other autoimmune diseases.

Autoantibody	Disease association
Adrenal cortex	
cytoplasmic	Addison's disease
	Cushing's syndrome
ACTH receptor	
blocking	Addison's disease
stimulating	Cushing's syndrome
Pituitary cells	Polyendocrine disease
Parathyroid: cytoplasmic	Hypoparathyroidism
Hypothalamus	Diabetes insipidus
Sperm	Male infertility
	Mumps orchitis
	Trauma; vasectomy
Ovary: steroid cells	Primary amenorrhoea
	Premature menopause

Fig. 4 Autoantibodies are found in most endocrine diseases, though not in all cases. Antibodies to sperm and to the ACTH receptor may be pathogenic; the others listed here are probably mainly of diagnostic and prognostic importance only.

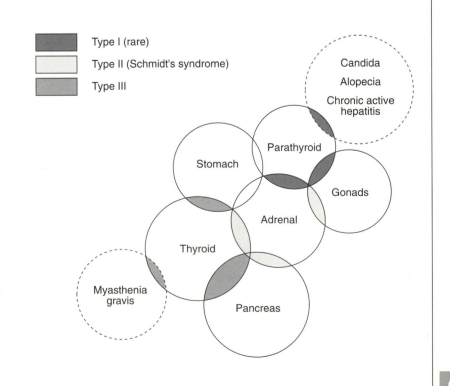

- Type I (rare)
- Type II (Schmidt's syndrome)
- Type III

Fig. 5 A striking feature of autoimmune endocrine diseases is the tendency for more than one to occur together in one patient (and also in relatives). Of the various overlaps shown in the figure, three patterns occur often enough to be recognized as distinct 'types' of polyendocrine syndrome, some of which are also associated with other autoimmune diseases or with abnormal responses to infection (shown in dotted lines). Like the individual diseases, these syndromes are often associated with HLA DR3, but many other genetic influences are clearly involved, and in some cases there may simply be cross-reaction between antigens from two or more organs.

Renal Disease

Of the renal causes of kidney failure (remember it can be pre- or post-renal as well!), a considerable proportion have an immunological basis. Indeed the kidney is one of the organs most susceptible to immune damage. Unfortunately the terminology of renal disease, already confusing because of the use of both clinical and histological classifications, is made worse by the addition of immunological terms intended to explain the cause of the pathology.

The clinical view

Clinicians think in terms of acute and chronic renal failure, acute nephritic syndrome, nephrotic syndrome, etc. A major cause of all of these conditions is **glomerulonephritis**, and the first two may also, but less commonly, be caused by damage to the tubules and interstitium (**'interstitial nephritis'**). The clinician will look to see if the renal disease is part of a more widespread *systemic* condition such as SLE, diabetes, infection, etc. The clinician is nowadays also expected to decide whether a patient with renal failure is a candidate for transplantation (see p. 51).

The pathologist's view

Pathologists classify what they see in renal biopsies or at post-mortem in terms of the *type* of cell affected (in the glomerulus: endothelium, epithelium, mesangium; in the tubules: distal, proximal; or in the interstitium), the *extent* of damage (focal, segmental, diffuse) and the *nature* of the lesion (proliferative, membranous, crescentic).

The immunologist's contribution

Two major breakthroughs have shed some light on the confusion. (1) The technique of **immunofluorescent staining** (see p. 93) demonstrated the presence of antibody in many cases in the diseased areas and (2) animal experiments showed that immune complexes formed during antibody responses to a variety of antigens could become deposited in the glomerulus, and also that antibody could be raised specifically against the glomerular basement membrane (GBM) (Fig. 1). On this basis, many cases of glomerulonephritis are now classified as either 'immune complex mediated' — which would be an example of type III hypersensitivity — or, rarely, mediated by anti-GBM antibodies, which are by definition autoantibodies (an example of type II hypersensitivity). However, there is also evidence of a role for **T cells and cytokines** in glomerulonephritis. In some cases of interstitial nephritis due to drugs, anti-tubular basement (TBM) antibodies are found.

What is the antigen?

A frustrating aspect of both immune complex disease and autoimmunity is that the triggering antigen can often not be identified. There are exceptions: immune complexes deposited during or after infection are presumed to contain antigens from the infectious organism, and sometimes this has in fact been proved (Fig. 2). In SLE, the complexes are predominantly anti-DNA, though it is not known why patients should make this autoantibody. Interstitial nephritis frequently follows the use of certain drugs (Fig. 3), and here the drug itself is probably modifying a TBM antigen or, alternatively, stimulating T-cell help for anti-TBM B cells. But in many cases, including the mysterious **IgA nephropathy** where IgA and complement are deposited in the mesangium, no inducing antigen has been demonstrated and a primary defect in IgA handling is suspected (Fig. 1).

Systemic diseases and the kidney

Immunological kidney disease is often part of a more widespread condition. As part of the vascular system, the glomerulus can be involved in **vasculitis** of any kind, often associated with **skin lesions** (Fig. 4). Anti-GBM antibodies often react with **lung basement membrane** too (Goodpasture's syndrome). The kidney is a common site of **amyloid** deposition, of both the 'light chain' and the 'serum amyloid A' type. Tubular damage is a serious complication of **myeloma.**

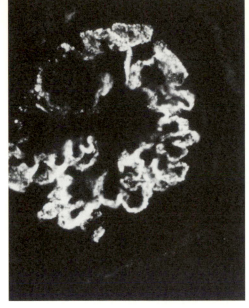

(a)

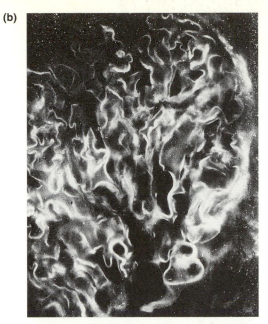

(b)

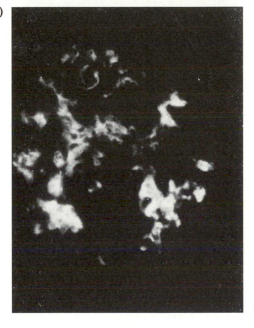

(c)

Fig. 1 Immunofluorescent demonstration of Ig deposition in the kidney. The same techniques can be used to show deposition of complement and (sometimes) antigen. **(a)** Immune complexes in the glomerulus from a case of membranous glomerulonephritis; the granular appearance is often referred to as 'lumpy-bumpy'. **(b)** A kidney from a case of Goodpasture's syndrome showing the linear deposition of anti-GBM antibody. **(c)** In this case of IgA nephropathy, IgA has been deposited exclusively in the mesangium.

Type	Specific organism
Virus	Hepatitis B (+ systemic vasculitis)
	CMV
	EBV
Bacteria	Streptococci (Gp A, β haemolytic)
	Strep. viridans (endocarditis)
	Staphylococci
	M. leprae
	T. pallidum
	Meningococci
Protozoa	*P. malariae* (nephrotic syndrome)
	P. falciparum
	Trypanosomes
	Toxoplasma gondii
Helminths	*Schistosoma mansoni, haematobium*
Foreign serum	(serum sickness)
Autoantigens	Antinuclear (e.g. DNA in SLE)
	Thyroglobulin

Fig. 2 Immune complexes are deposited in the glomerulus in a variety of infectious diseases. Streptococcal throat infection and quartan malaria are among the commonest worldwide.

Type	Specific drug
Antibiotics	Penicillin
	Methicillin
	Ampicillin
	Sulphonamides
	Rifampicin
Anti-inflammatory	Phenylbutazone
	Ibuprofen
	Gold
	Allopurinol
	Aspirin
Diuretics	Thiazides
	Frusemide
Anticonvulsants	Phenytoin
	Phenobarbitone
Immunosuppressive	Azathioprine

Fig. 3 A variety of drugs can cause tubular damage by binding to the TBM and inducing anti-TBM antibody or cell-mediated damage.

Vasculitis	SLE
	Polyarteritis nodosa
	Wegener's granulomatosis
	Henoch–Schonlein purpura
	Temporal arteritis
	Serum sickness
	Rheumatoid arthritis
Amyloid	
Myeloma	
Goodpasture's syndrome (plus lung)	
Diabetes	
Systemic sclerosis	

Fig. 4 The kidney is often involved in systemic diseases, especially those in which blood vessels are the target. Many or all of these may be caused by immune complex deposition and as well as the kidney, lesions in the skin and lung are common.

66

The Eye and Nervous System

The eye

The eye is susceptible to infection and to various hypersensitivity reactions, and is also involved in several systemic immunological diseases.

- **Infection.** The anterior eye is normally protected by tears, which contain **lysozyme** and **IgA** antibody. Nevertheless, conjunctivitis and infections of the uveal tract (iris, ciliary body, choroid) can be caused by a variety of organisms, including several of tropical importance (Fig. 1).
- **Hypersensitivity.** This may be mainly localized (e.g. to the eye and nose in hay fever) but is more often part of a more widespread condition (Fig. 2). Uveitis is surprisingly often associated with arthritis, the common feature probably being deposition of immune complexes (type III hypersensitivity).
- **Immunological diseases.** The cornea, having no blood or lymph drainage, can be replaced by an allograft, although about 5% of corneal grafts do become vascularized and are rejected (see pp. 51 & 83). Exposure of eye antigens to the immune system, e.g. after penetrating injury, can cause an autoimmune uveitis affecting the normal eye (**sympathetic ophthalmia**), and a similar effect can follow lens replacement.

The nervous system

The blood–brain barrier

The brain has its own dendritic antigen-presenting/phagocytic cells (**microglia**) but because of the tight endothelial junctions and the lack of lymphatics the brain is normally excluded from blood-borne cells and molecules (e.g. lymphocytes, antibody). Therefore, the presence of cells in the CSF usually indicates infection, while antibody is often a sign of multiple sclerosis (see below).

Infection of the meninges is usually bacterial, while the brain and spinal cord are especially susceptible to viral infection (encephalitis, myelitis). Figure 3 lists the important organisms. Note that several of these are opportunists, CNS infection being much commoner in immunodeficient patients. A number of rare but important neurological diseases are thought to be late complications of infection, notably **subacute sclerosing pan-encephalitis**, occurring many years after measles, and possibly the fatigue and muscle weakness of the 'post-viral syndrome'.

Demyelination and multiple sclerosis

The myelin sheath is vital to the function of neurones, acting as an insulator, and destruction of myelin has drastic effects on nerve conduction. The most important demyelinating disease is **multiple sclerosis** which affects about six people per 10 000 in the UK and up to three per 1000 in some more northern areas, with an age peak around 30. The characteristic feature is the plaque, in which T and B lymphocytes and macrophages accumulate and myelin is intermittently but progressively destroyed (Fig. 4). The CSF contains lymphocytes and, on electrophoresis, oligoclonal bands of IgG. Demyelination can also occur in peripheral nerves (e.g. the **Guillain–Barré syndrome**), but here recovery is usually complete.

Autoimmune neurological diseases

The muscle weakness and fatiguability of **myasthenia gravis** is due to an autoimmune destruction of acetylcholine receptors at the nerve–muscle junction (Fig. 5). Since (1) the symptoms can be passively transferred from mother to newborn, (2) IgG anti-receptor antibody is found in the serum and at sites of receptor destruction and (3) its removal (by plasmapheresis) can temporarily relieve the symptoms, it is considered that the antibody is in fact the cause of the disease. There is a strong association with HLA B8/DR3 and with thymic changes, including thymoma.

The brain is often involved, usually only mildly, in **systemic lupus erythematosus**.

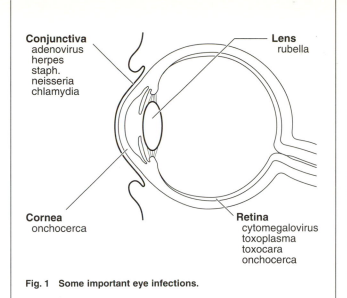

Fig. 1 Some important eye infections.

Conjunctiva
adenovirus
herpes
staph.
neisseria
chlamydia

Lens
rubella

Cornea
onchocerca

Retina
cytomegalovirus
toxoplasma
toxocara
onchocerca

Eye structure affected	Disease
Conjunctiva	Hay fever (nose)
Uveal tract	Ankylosing spondylitis (arthritis)
	Reiter's syndrome (arthritis, urethritis)
	Rheumatoid arthritis (arthritis, anaemia etc.)
	Sjögren's syndrome (arthritis, salivary gland)
	Stevens–Johnson syndrome (skin, mouth)
	Behcet's disease (arthritis, mucosal ulcers)
	Crohn's; ulcerative colitis (intestine)
	Sarcoidosis (multi-system granulomata)
	Vasculitis (SLE, polyarteritis nodosa)
	Pemphigoid (skin)
Retro-orbital muscles	Graves' disease (hyperthyroidism)

Fig. 2 Inflammatory eye disease, of presumed immunological origin, is a feature of many systemic diseases.

Condition	Infective cause
Meningitis	*Neisseria meningitidis*
	Haemophilus influenzae
	Strep. pneumoniae
	Syphilis
	Tuberculosis
	(any septicaemia)
	Herpes simplex; zoster
	Measles, mumps
	HIV
	Cryptococci*
Encephalomyelitis	Herpes simplex; zoster; CMV*
	Poliomyelitis; ECHO; Coxsackie
	Rabies
	Measles (SSPE)
	Malaria (*P. falciparum* only)
	Trypanosomes (African)
	Toxoplasma*
	Prion diseases
	Creutzfeld–Jacob disease
	Kuru
	Alzheimer's disease
Peripheral neuritis	Leprosy
	Diphtheria
	HIV
Cysts and abscesses	Amoeba
	Tapeworms

Fig. 3 A number of organisms can infect the CNS, especially in immunodeficient patients (*).

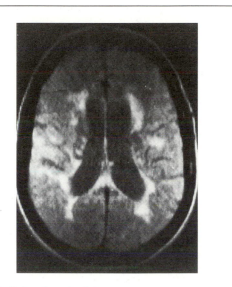

Fig. 4 **Multiple sclerosis.** Extensive demyelination in the cerebral hemispheres shown in an MRI scan.

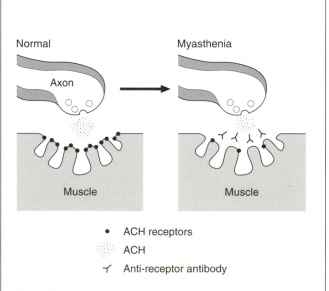

Normal   Myasthenia

Axon

Muscle   Muscle

- ●   ACH receptors
- ⦂   ACH
- ⅄   Anti-receptor antibody

Fig. 5 **Myasthenia gravis.** Antibody to the acetylcholine receptor on the muscle end-plate, together with complement, leads to destruction of the receptors and an inadequate signal for muscle contraction.

Skin Disease

In its role as outer lining of the body, the skin is exposed to enormous doses of foreign antigens which, if they do penetrate, are usually presented via epidermal Langerhans cells to T cells both locally and in the regional lymph nodes. Therefore, it can be considered an immunological organ in its own right. In addition, the skin can be the target of a remarkable range of immunopathological disorders, including examples of all the four classical types of hypersensitivity (Fig.1), while an immunological element is suspected in a number of idiopathic skin diseases.

Dermatitis, urticaria and eczema

The most clear-cut example of hypersensitivity to an external antigen is **allergic contact dermatitis** in which the changes typical of type IV hypersensitivity (T-cell-mediated, see p. 45) are induced by a range of chemicals (Fig. 2). By contrast, most cases of **urticaria** are due to a type I reaction ('allergic'; see p. 45) associated with raised IgE, mast-cell degranulation and increased vascular permeability. Not all urticarial swelling is allergic; for example **hereditary angioedema** is due to a genetic deficiency of the normal inhibitor of C1 esterase, resulting in uncontrolled kinin generation with oedema in the skin and intestine (see p. 54).

The most puzzling type of dermatitis is **atopic eczema** in which eczematous changes are seen in association with raised IgE and a family history of eczema, asthma, hay fever and food allergy (Fig. 3). Here the defect may be in the regulatory activities of T cells.

Autoimmunity

Type II (cytotoxic) hypersensitivity is the basis of the **bullous** ('blistering') diseases (Fig. 4) in which autoantibodies and complement are found at various sites in the skin. The most serious of these, **pemphigus**, is a 'true' autoimmune disease because serum from a patient can transfer the skin changes to a newborn infant or an experimental animal (the same is true for Graves' disease and myasthenia gravis). Treatment is based on combinations of immunosuppressive drugs: steroids, azathioprine and cyclosporine.

Immune complexes and vasculitis

Like the kidney (see p. 65) the skin is frequently involved in diseases where antigen-antibody complexes are formed in the circulation: Gell and Coombs type III hypersensitivity. The different syndromes are thought to be due to differences in the size of the complex, the class of antibody, the site of production and local conditions — blood vessel size, inflammation, etc. Sometimes other organs are involved too, so that vasculitis is a component of a number of important systemic diseases (Fig. 5). Note however that not all vasculitis is due to complexes; sometimes lymphocytic infiltration around the blood vessel is the only sign of immunological involvement, and in some cases PMN may become unusually destructive to vessel walls because of the action of cytokines or autoantibodies.

Infection and immunodeficiency

Of the common skin rashes, some are due to straightforward infection (e.g. with staphylococci, streptococci, chickenpox) while others are the result of an immune response (e.g. measles). A healthy skin evidently depends on healthy cell-mediated immunity, because a number of skin diseases are only seen in patients with immunodeficiency affecting the T cells (Fig. 6). In line with this is the fact that the rejection of an incompatible skin graft appears to be carried out exclusively by T cell-mediated responses, whereas with organs like the kidney, antibodies are also involved in rejection (see p. 51).

Skin disease	Hypersensitivity type	Mechanisms involved
Urticaria	I	IgE; mast cells; histamine
Bullous diseases	II	Autoantibody to skin components; complement
Vasculitis	III	Immune complexes; PMN; complement
Allergic contact dermatitis	IV	T cells; cytokines

Fig. 1 Hypersensitivity reactions of all types can show up as skin conditions.

Nickel, chromium
Rubber components
Epoxy resins
Drugs: sulphonamides, neomycin
Drugs and plant products activated by sunlight
Poison ivy, garden flowers
Cosmetics; lanolin

Fig. 2 **Contact sensitivity (dermatitis) can be due to a variety of occupation-related antigens which penetrate the skin, bind to proteins or cells and stimulate T cells.** Note than unlike the majority of antigens, most of them are not proteins. Diagnosis is by delayed (patch) skin testing.

Allergy-related
House-dust mite allergy
Food allergies (milk, egg, fish, nuts, etc.)
Raised serum IgE
Positive skin prick tests

Immunodeficiency-related
Depressed delayed skin reactions
Susceptibility to viruses (e.g. herpes, warts)
Association with T cell deficiencies

Fig. 3 **The immunological findings in atopic eczema suggest a deficiency of T cells,** including those that normally regulate IgE production.

	Pemphigus	Pemphigoid	Herpes gestationis	Dermatitis herpetiformis
Immunofluorescent staining pattern	IgG, C3 Intercellular cement 'honeycomb'	IgG, C3 Dermo-epidermal junction	(IgG), C3 as pemphigoid	IgA, (C3) Dermal papillae 'granular'
Other associations	Drugs	Drugs	Pregnancy	Coeliac disease
HLA association	DR 4		DR 3, 4	B8, DR 3
Treatment	Steroids, azathioprine	Steroids	Steroids	Gluten-free diet

Fig. 4 **Four rare but potentially serious 'bullous' skin diseases are associated with autoantibodies to skin components.** The inducing agents are usually not known but they may follow exposure to drugs or, in the case of dermatitis herpetiformis, wheat foods.

Type	Specific disease
Vasculitis	SLE (+ joints, kidney, CNS)
	Discoid lupus (skin only)
	Polyarteritis nodosa (+ lungs, kidney)
	Wegener's granulomatosis (+ lungs, kidney)
	Henoch–Schonlein purpura (+ kidney)
	Erythema nodosum (+ joints)
	Serum sickness (+ joints)
	Temporal arteritis (+ eyes)
	Erythema multiforme (+ mouth, eyes)
	Cryoglobulinaemia (+ kidney, joints)
Idiopathic	Systemic sclerosis (scleroderma) (+ gut, heart, joints, kidney, CNS, etc.)
	Psoriasis (+ joints)

Fig. 5 **The skin is involved in many systemic diseases, often together with other organs** (see also p. 65). Damage to blood vessels by immune complexes is thought to be the commonest underlying cause.

Patient	Pathology	Examples
Normal	Cytopathic virus	Smallpox, chickenpox
	Virus-induced hypertrophy	Warts
	Immune response to virus	Measles rash
	Bacterial toxin	Scarlet fever (streptococci), impetigo (strep, staphylococci),
	Immune response to bacteria	Typhoid rash
	Fungal growth	Tinea (ringworm)
	Protozoal growth	Cutaneous leishmaniasis
Immunodeficient	T cell deficiency (especially AIDS)	Candida, warts Molluscum contagiosum, Kaposi's sarcoma
	Wiskott–Aldrich syndrome	Eczema
	Graft-v-host disease	Exfoliative dermatitis

Fig. 6 **The skin is involved in many infectious diseases, of which some representative examples are shown.**

Connective Tissue Diseases (1)

Diseases of the musculoskeletal system are relatively common and result in the loss of many work-hours. *Autoimmunity* plays an important role in the pathogenesis of many of these (see p. 47 for discussion of the mechanisms). For convenience, we consider here the inflammatory diseases mainly affecting the joints and spine. Those with more widespread effects are described on the following pages.

Rheumatoid arthritis (RA)

RA is the commonest of the immunologically-mediated joint diseases, affecting up to 1% of the population with a 3:1 preponderance of F:M and with some association with HLA-Dw4 (see p. 83). The diagnostic criteria for RA are shown in Figure 1. Although it mainly affects the synovial joints, extra-articular manifestations are frequent and usually develop as the disease progresses (Fig. 2). **Rheumatoid factor (RF)** is defined as an autoantibody to the Fc region of IgG. RF is mainly of the IgM class and of limited diagnostic value since it only occurs in 70% of RA patients but is found in patients with other rheumatic diseases (see p. 73). However, a persistently high titre of RF does signify more aggressive disease. Low titres of antinuclear antibodies are found in 30% of RA patients. C3 and C4 levels are usually normal or elevated whilst C-reactive protein levels are elevated (see p. 9). Hypergammaglobulinaemia is unusual. Amyloidosis occurs in at least 12% of patients with RA.

Figure 3 shows the villous nature of RA synovial tissue which becomes infiltrated with macrophages, T cells (mainly CD4) and plasma cells (many secreting RF). Cytokines and immune complexes (through hypersensitivity type III reactions, p. 45) within the joint are thought to contribute to damage to the cartilage and bone erosion (Fig. 4). T cells (through type IV hypersensitivity reactions) are also thought to contribute to this chronic inflammatory disease.

The aetiology of RA is unknown but viruses, such as Epstein–Barr virus and parvovirus, and bacteria, especially mycobacteria, have been implicated. Microorganisms have, however, not been isolated from affected joints.

Seronegative arthritides

By definition, patients with these diseases lack RF. Unlike patients with RA the majority of patients with seronegative arthritides do not progress to chronic peripheral joint disease. (Ankylosing spondylitis is an exception.) Seronegative arthritides in which an association with infectious microorganisms has been described include:

- **Ankylosing spondylitis (AS)**. This affects the spine and sacroiliac joints, mainly in men, with a frequency of 0.4%. Complications include iritis, uveitis and peripheral arthritis. HLA typing for B27 is used in diagnosis and this HLA has the highest association with any disease to date (see HLA, p. 83). Antibodies to *Klebsiella* are raised in AS and their reactivity with HLA-B27 supports an antigenic mimicry hypothesis for autoantibody production in this disease. This hypothesis does not , however, explain the localized nature of the disease in the sacroiliac joints and spinal-ligamentous insertions.
- **Reiter's disease**. This 'reactive arthritis' is thought to be a sequel of non-gonococcal genitourinary infections (*Chlamydia* or *Campylobacter*) or bowel infections by *Shigella* or *Yersinia*. As with AS, there is a strong association with HLA-B27. Clinical features of Reiter's disease usually include conjunctivitis and a skin rash (see pp. 67 & 69).

Seronegative arthritides in which no association with microorganisms has been found to date are listed in Fig. 5.

Infectious arthritis

Infective agents alone (e.g. staphylococci, gonococci, TB) or as immune complexes (e.g. streptococci, rubella and mumps) can cause arthritis. The arthritis of rheumatic fever may also, like the myocarditis, be due to autoantibodies triggered by cross-reacting streptococcal antigens.

Juvenile arthritis

The classification of juvenile arthritis is shown in Figure 6. This is by definition an arthritis which occurs in children of 16 and under. Amyloidosis is an occasional complication in this condition.

Criteria	Definition
Morning stiffness	Lasting >1 hour
Arthritis-3 or more joint areas	Soft tissue swelling or fluid
Arthritis of hand joints	In wrist, MCP or PIP joints
Symmetric arthritis	Simultaneous joint involvement of areas on both sides of body
Rheumatoid nodules	Subcutaneous, over bony prominences
Serum RF	Elevated by assay showing < 5% in control subjects
Radiographic changes	Typical on posteroanterior hand and wrist, must include erosions or unequivocal bony decalcification

Fig. 1 American Rheumatism Association revised criteria for diagnosis of RA (1988). MCP, metocarpophalangeal; PIP, proximal interphalangeal.

Rheumatoid nodules (skin, lung)
Anaemia
Vasculitis
Keratoconjunctivitis (secondary SS)
Sicca syndrome
Neutropenia (Felty's)
Pericarditis
Pleurisy
Fibrosing alveolitis
Carpal tunnel syndrome

Fig. 2 Extra-articular disease in RA.

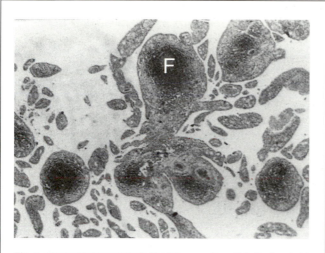

Fig. 3 Marked hypertrophy in the RA synovium. Note the lymphoid follicles (F).

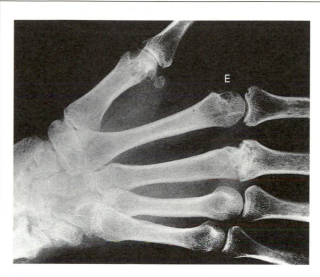

Fig. 4 X-ray of the hand of a patient with RA. Note the narrowing of joint spaces and bony erosions (E).

Disease	Frequency
Psoriatic arthritis	2% of patients with psoriasis
Relapsing polychondritis	Rare; most patients have episodes of non-symmetrical arthritis
Behçet's disease	Multisystem disorder: 45% of patients develop arthritis; 15% present with it.
Scleroderma	25% of patients develop arthritis, often early in disease

Fig. 5 Other seronegative arthritides.

Type	Frequency	Characteristics
JRA	(10%)	Features of adult RA, erosive, RF positive
JAS	(15%)	RF seronegative
JCA		RF seronegative
Pauciarticular	(50%)	< 5 joints affected, associated with iridocyclitis
Polyarticular	(10%)	> 5 joints affected
Systemic	(15%)	Young onset severe systemic disease

Fig. 6 Classification of juvenile arthritis. JRA, juvenile RA; JAS, juvenile ankylosing spondylitis; JCA, juvenile chronic arthritis.

Connective Tissue Diseases (2)

Systemic lupus erythematosus (SLE)

SLE is a multi-organ autoimmune disease with a prevalence of 0.5–1.5 per 1000 in the general population depending on geographical location and race (black > Chinese > caucasian). It occurs mainly in young women (20–40 years old). Patients may have a rash across the cheeks and nose (said to be wolf-like, hence *lupus*, latin) (Fig. 1) but typically present with arthritis. By comparison with rheumatoid arthritis (RA), usually many body systems are also affected (Fig. 2). A comparison of some distinguishing clinical criteria for SLE and RA is shown in Figure 3. Patients virtually all have anti-nuclear antibodies (ANA), most have hypergammaglobulinaemia, antibodies to double stranded DNA (dsDNA) and *reduced* C3 and C4 levels, particularly when the disease is active. Unlike patients with RA, only a quarter have RF. Up to 40% of patients have antiphospholipid antibodies including the **'lupus anticoagulant'** (see p. 75). Tissue damage is mainly due to deposition of immune complexes (*type III hypersensitivity*). The aetiology of SLE is multifactorial with hormonal, genetic and environmental factors contributing. Renal disease and bacterial/viral infections are the main causes of death in SLE patients, the latter problems being largely secondary to immunosuppressive therapy. **Drug-induced lupus** may occur in certain individuals and this has many of the features of SLE but with less renal disease. Drugs responsible include hydralazine and procainamide (see p. 88).

Polymyositis (PM)

In this disease which presents with proximal muscle weakness, 40% of the patients develop a mild peripheral arthritis, usually transient and non-erosive. The majority of the patients have evidence of increased serum muscle enzymes and abnormal electromyography and muscle biopsies. A subset of patients also have skin lesions (**dermatomyositis**). Polymyositis can also be associated with RA, SLE, Sjögren's syndrome or systemic sclerosis ('secondary'). In recent years, a number of disease specific antibodies, e.g. Jo-1, directed against tRNA synthetase enzymes have been identified.

Systemic sclerosis (scleroderma)

Systemic sclerosis (SCL) can affect the skin, musculoskeletal system, blood vessels and many other organs (see p. 69). The severest form is life-threatening (**progressive** systemic sclerosis). The main characteristics of the disease are shown in Figure 4.

Sjögren's syndrome (SS)

Primary SS is characterized by keratoconjunctivitis sicca (dry eyes) and xerostomia (dry mouth) – the sicca complex. It may also be **secondary** to RA and other autoimmune diseases. By itself, the 'sicca complex' in SS is not life-threatening but up to 13% of patients progress to lymphoma. It is this, RA and other autoimmune diseases which provide the main clinical problems. The 'sicca complex' is thought to be due to damage to the salivary, lachrimal and other exocrine glands by a CD4$^+$ T lymphocyte infiltrate (see p. 61). Characteristically, patients have serum antibodies to the ribonucleoprotein complex **La (SS-B)** and/or **Ro (SS-A)** and these are of diagnostic value. Treatment is usually symptomatic.

Mixed connective tissue disease (MCTD)

A small group of patients have the clinical and laboratory features of SLE, polymyositis and systemic sclerosis which can occur simultaneously or sequentially and are said to have **'overlap syndrome'** (Fig. 5). Whether or not it is clinically useful to define a patient group in this way is debateable especially since it may represent a prodromal state leading to one or other of the disease trio.

Treatment of connective tissue diseases

Like treatment of most of the other autoimmune diseases, therapy involves alleviation of the chronic inflammation by drugs, including steroids and immunosuppressives, as shown in Figure 6. Mechanisms of action of these drugs are discussed in 'Drugs and the immune system' (p. 87).

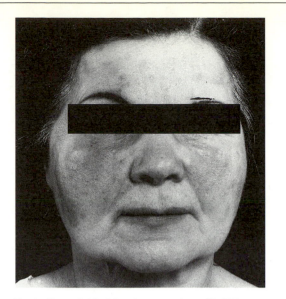

Fig. 1 'Butterfly' facial rash on a patient with SLE.

Organ	Presentation
Joints	Arthritis/arthralgia
Heart	Pericarditis
Blood	Anaemia/leukopenia
	Vasculitis
Lungs	Pleurisy/pericarditis
Kidneys	Nephrotic syndrome
Skin	Cutaneous lesions (e.g. facial rash)
Brain	Neuropsychiatric problems

Fig. 2 Organ systems affected in SLE.

Characteristic	RA	SLE
Onset (yr)	30–60	20–40
Sex ratio (F:M)	3:1	9:1
Facial rash	–	+
Lung involvement	FA	Pleurisy
Pericarditis	rare	+
Nodules	+	–
Proteinuria	rare	+
Joint erosions	+	–
Peripheral neuropathy	+	–/+
Neuropsychiatric problems	–	+
Vasculitis	+/–	+

Fig. 3 Clinical comparisons between RA and SLE. FA, fibrosing alveolitis.

Clinical/laboratory findings	Patients (%)
Elevated rheumatoid factors	25–33
Serum immununoglobulins raised	25–50
Anti-nuclear antibodies	30–95
Progressive systemic sclerosis	10
CREST syndrome (**C**alcinosis,	70–97
Raynaud's phenomenon,	
Esophageal dysmotility, **S**clerodactyly, **T**elangiectasia)	

Fig. 4 Systemic sclerosis.

Disease	Drugs
RA	
First line	NSAIDs including asprin, indomethacin, ibuprofen
Second line*	Sulphasalazine, gold, penicillamine
Third line*	Azathioprine, methotrexate, cyclophosphamide**
SLE, MCTD, SCL, PM	Steroids e.g. prednisone Cytotoxics e.g. azathioprine Cyclophosphamide

Fig. 6 Main drugs used to treat connective tissue diseases. NSAIDs, non-steroidal anti-inflammatory drugs; * requires monitoring bone-marrow depression; ** used for systemic complications.

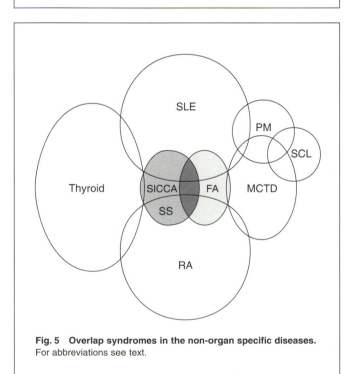

Fig. 5 Overlap syndromes in the non-organ specific diseases. For abbreviations see text.

Blood Diseases

The mature cells of the haemopoietic system are vulnerable to antibodies, including autoantibodies. Other immune diseases of the blood are associated with antibodies to erythroid progenitor cells or clotting factors. Immunoproliferative disorders are described on page 85.

Immune anaemias

- **Autoimmune haemolytic anaemias (AIHA)** can be primary or secondary to other diseases (Fig. 1). Damage to mature erythrocytes (RBC) is mediated mainly through antibodies and complement. Antibodies are detected by the antiglobulin (**Coombs'**) test. The different types and causes of AIHA are shown in Figure 2. The warm antibody haemolytic anaemias (HA) are polyclonal and mainly directed to **rhesus** type antigens whilst the cold antibodies can be monoclonal and react mainly with **I antigens**. In the warm antibody HA, the RBC are mainly removed by the red pulp phagocytic system of the spleen. The cold antibody HA are divided into the cold haemagglutinin diseases (CHAD) and the rarer paroxysmal cold haemoglobulinuria (PCH). Unlike patients with the cold type diseases who have intravascular haemolysis, those with the warm HA respond reasonably well to steroids and splenectomy.
- **Aplastic anaemia** and **red cell aplasia** can be immunological. Erythropoeisis can be disrupted by IgG autoantibodies directed at erythrocyte progenitors (acquired red cell aplasia).
- **Non-autoimmune haemolytic anaemias** can be caused by antibodies directed either to the major blood groups (see below) or maternal antibodies to fetal red cell antigens, the most common being rhesus D antigen in **haemolytic anaemia of the newborn** (see p. 46).
- **Megaloblastic anaemias** occur when autoantibodies to intrinsic factor result in pernicious anaemia by blocking vitamin B_{12} absorption (see pp. 45, 47 & 61).

Immune neutropenias

The immune neutropenias can be idiopathic or secondary to SLE and other immune complex diseases (Fig. 3). Like the haemolytic anaemias and thrombocytopenias, they can be caused by autoantibodies, alloantibodies and drugs. Removal of the drug results in clinical improvement. Treatment is mainly with prednisolone or (still experimental) intravenous immunoglobulins.

Immune thrombocytopenias

These diseases can also be primary (idiopathic) or secondary with an acute or chronic course. Secondary disease is more frequently chronic and can occur with SLE and lymphoproliferative disorders including non-Hodgkin's lymphoma and CLL. Figure 4 lists major differences between acute and chronic **idiopathic thrombocytopenia purpura (ITP)**. Transmission of IgG platelet autoantibodies across the placenta of mothers with chronic ITP or with alloantibodies due to sensitization by paternal platelet antigens, results in neonatal thrombocytopenia. The mechanisms involved in causing drug-induced thrombocytopenia are similar to those for the drug-induced anaemias (see Fig. 1). Implicated drugs include quinine, quinidine and sedormid. Removal of the drug results in clinical improvement.

Immune coagulation disorders

Prolonged activated partial thromboplastin time (APPT) may be the result of antibodies to a number of components of the clotting system. Antibodies to **factor VIII** in haemophiliacs are the most common anticoagulant factors (Fig. 5) but antibodies can occur spontaneously (but rarely) in SLE patients, patients with lymphoproliferative disorders and elderly patients without demonstrable underlying disease. **'Lupus anticoagulant'** antibodies and **anti-cardiolipin** antibodies are also clinically important (see SLE, p. 73)

Blood incompatibility complications

The numerous complications of blood group polymorphisms are summarized in Figure 6.

Primary (idiopathic) > 50%
Secondary to:
  SLE/RA
  CLL/non-Hodgkin's lymphoma
  Infection: mycoplasma, EBV
  Drug treatment

Fig. 1 Primary and secondary AIHA. CLL, chronic lymphocytic leukaemia; EBV, Epstein–Barr virus.

Type of anaemia	%	Damage due to
Warm antibody	70	Mainly IgG; opsonization and phagocytosis
Cold antibody	18	Mainly IgM, except PCH (unusual IgG); intravascular haemolysis related to cold
Drug-induced, e.g. penicillin, α-methyldopa	12	Antibodies to adsorbed drug Attachment of IC (drug /IgG) Autoantibodies to RBC (rhesus ag)

Fig. 2 The main causes of the autoimmune haemolytic anaemias: IC, immune complexes; PCH, paroxysmal cold haemoglobinuria.

Primary (idiopathic)
Secondary to:
  Immune complex disease, e.g. SLE, Sjögren's syndrome; RA – Felty's syndrome (splenomegaly with high titre RF)
  Drugs e.g. aminopyrine

Fig. 3 Classification of immune neutropenias.

Acute ITP	Chronic ITP
Onset during childhood	20–50 years old
M = F	F:M = 3:1
Sometimes prior infection	No association with infection
Variable levels of platelets	Variable levels of platelets
Spontaneous resolution	Resolution rare
Duration short	Duration months to years
No treatment	Treated with corticosteroids ± splenectomy

Fig. 4 A comparison of acute and chronic ITP.

Antibodies	Patient group	Comments
Factor VIII	Severe haemophiliacs	Up to 20% patients receiving blood products
'Lupus anti-coagulant' (LA)	SLE	Up to 40% of patients; paradoxically cause thrombosis
Anti-cardiolipin (anti-phospholipid)	Primary anti-phospholipid antibody syndrome	Same as LA? Give false positives in syphilis test

Fig. 5 Immune coagulation disorders.

Source of incompatibility	Clinical manifestations
Transfusion	Natural isoagglutinins of the ABO system make matching essential; transfusions sensitize against blood group antigens especially rhesus D; recipients pre-screened for rare pre-existing antibodies by agglutination for IgM 'complete' and IgG 'incomplete' antibodies (indirect antiglobulin test — Coombs' test); an ABO mismatch can cause an immediate reaction with massive haemolysis due to IgM and complement
Multiple transfusions	Despite careful screening, occasional delayed reactions can occur; these may be due to HLA antigens
Haemolytic disease of the newborn	Paternal rhesus (mainly D) antigens can sensitize a rhesus negative mother, giving rise to antibodies that can affect subsequent babies; it can be prevented successfully in 99% of cases by injection of the mother with rhesus D antibodies within 48 hours of birth or during delivery

Fig. 6 Blood incompatibility complications.

Infectious Disease

Basic and pathological background

First, refresh your memory of the types of infectious organism, how they are normally dealt with (p. 37) and how they try to escape (p. 39). Then recall the ways they can cause disease (p. 49) and how different types of immunodeficiency can predispose to infection (p. 53). Here we are concerned with some of the clinical aspects of common infections which have an immunological significance.

Diagnosis

This is often made by clinical or microbiological observation, but lymphocytes are more observant than the sharpest eye and their responses can provide a wealth of detailed information about microorganisms. This works two ways: if the organism is available (e.g. bacteria in the faeces or a throat swab), standard antibodies can be used to identify it. Alternatively if the organism is not detectable, its presence can be deduced by looking in the blood for antibodies made during infection or by examining the response of T cells to various standard antigens, either in culture or by skin test. Details of some of these tests will be found on pages 91–94.

The clinical pattern

Very acute symptoms, coming on within hours of exposure, are likely to be due to toxins, and antibodies to these, if available, can be life-saving. At the opposite end of the spectrum, symptoms that develop over weeks or months would make the clinician think in terms of chronic infection; about 30% of PUO (pyrexia of unknown origin) is due to infection, more so in children. Persistent infections such as TB, fungi, worms, because of the difficulty in eliminating the organism, may induce strong cell-mediated responses leading to severe pathology (granuloma, fibrosis). A fluctuating disease pattern, with regular remissions and relapses, is typical of organisms that can vary their antigens rapidly; brucellosis, relapsing fever (borrelia) and sleeping sickness (trypanosomiasis) are examples. Antigenic variation on a slower time scale shows up in the lack of immunity to repeated attacks of what appears to be the same disease (common cold, influenza). Figure 1 shows some typical patterns of infection and immunity.

The immunocompromised patient

Such patients are more common than they used to be because of (1) immunosuppressive drug treatment for transplants, etc., (2) better diagnosis and care of primary immunodeficiency and (3) **AIDS**. Therefore opportunistic infections are on the increase (Fig. 2) and these can pose serious therapeutic problems. There are two approaches: (1) correction of the immunological defect where possible and (2) chemotherapy, often requiring novel compounds.

One should also remember that with respect to infections not often encountered by man, such as the zoonoses, we are all to some extent immunocompromised, since our immune system has not been forced to evolve effective defences against them. Some of them are among the most dangerous infections known (Fig. 3).

A third category of unusual infections is those acquired in hospital (nosocomial). Here the already high incidence of infection is made worse by crowding, surgical procedures and, most dangerous of all, resistance to antibiotics. The concept of 'hospital staphylococci' is a chilling reminder of the risk. The combination of immunosuppression and hospitalization that occurs following bone marrow transplantation (see also p. 53) can give rise to particularly dangerous infections (Fig. 4).

Infection and immunity in the tropics

Inhabitants of the tropics have to bear the double burden of (1) frequent malnutrition, which can severely compromise the immune system and (2) a range of organisms restricted to the tropics, most notably parasitic protozoa and worms (Fig. 5). Unfortunately these are some of the most difficult organisms for even the intact immune system to deal with; chemotherapy is not always effective and vaccines are currently unavailable. Since most of these diseases affect children as well as adults, tropical infectious disease can reasonably be considered the world's number one health problem.

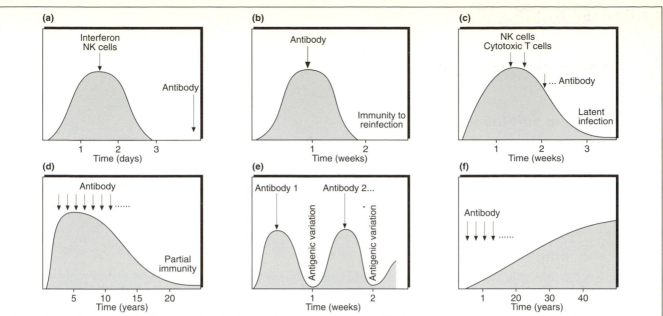

Fig. 1 **The pattern of infection is often determined by the type and effectiveness of the immune response.** Some examples are **(a)** common cold; **(b)** streptococcal pneumonia; **(c)** infectious mononucleosis; **(d)** malaria: **(e)** relapsing fever; **(f)** syphilis. Shaded areas indicate the presence of the infectious agent (and usually symptoms). Arrows indicate the principal immune mechanisms.

Type	Specific organisms
Primary	
Affecting myeloid cells	Bacteria (staph), fungi (*Aspergillus**)
Affecting complement	Bacteria (*Neisseria*: lytic pathway)
Affecting antibody	Bacteria, fungi, enteroviruses
Affecting T cells	Viruses, TB, fungi, protozoa
Secondary	
Splenectomy	Capsulated bacteria (*Strep. pneumoniae*), *Babesia**
Leukaemias	Bacteria, fungi
Immunosuppressive drugs steroids cytotoxics	
AIDS	Fungi (pneumocystis*), *Candida**, Toxoplasma*, *Mycobacteria* (atypical*), *Cryptosporidium*, HSV, CMV*

Fig. 2 **Patterns of infection in the immuno-compromised host vary somewhat with the cause of the immunodeficiency.** Organisms of major importance are shown in brackets. *These 'opportunistic' organisms are only pathogenic in immunodeficient patients. For further details of the situation in AIDS, see p. 81.

Organism	Direct contact	Food/water	Insect or animal bite	Inhalation
Viruses	Marburg*	Lassa*	Yellow fever* Dengue* Rabies*	Psittacosis
Bacteria	Anthrax *Brucella* *Leptospira**	*Brucella* *Salmonella* Tuberculosis *Listeria*	Plague* Typhus* Lyme disease Relapsing fever *Pasteurella*	Anthrax Q fever Tuberculosis
Fungi			Blastomycosis	*Histoplasma*
Protozoa		*Giardia* *Toxoplasma* *Cryptosporidium*	*Leishmania** Trypanosomiasis*	
Worms		Tapeworms		

Fig. 3 **Infections acquired by man from animals ('zoonoses') often have unusual features.** Obviously neither vaccine campaigns nor public health measures are likely to remove the reservoir of infection; at best a vaccine may protect the individual. They are usually better adapted to their natural host than to man, so that some of them (*) are acute, severe and often fatal.

Time after transplant	Immunological defect	Major infections
First 2–4 weeks	Marrow aplasia No PMN No lymphocytes	Bacteria: staphylococci, Gram-negative Fungi: candida, pneumocystis Viruses: HSV
After 4 weeks	PMN present (but function ↓) Lymphocytes: CD4 ↓ NK cells ↓ Ig ↓	Viruses: CMV* Fungi: *Aspergillus* Protozoa: *Toxoplasma*
3 months – 1 year	CD4/CD8 ratio ↓ IgG ↓	Capsulated bacteria
Graft-v-host disease	Spleen ↓ Macrophages ↓ IgG ↓, IgA ↓ CD8 T cells (donor)	Capsulated bacteria *Haemophilus* Skin rashes, diarrhoea, hepatitis

Fig. 4 **The post-transplant period is always a dangerous one because of infection.** This is especially true after bone marrow transplantation because of the very strong immunosuppression required, plus the risk of GVH disease.
* Of all the common infections, CMV carries the highest mortality — up to 80% in some series.

Infection	Immunity	Immunopathology
Viruses		
Yellow fever	Good vaccine	
Dengue		DIC; Enhancing antibody
Bacteria		
Plague	Vaccine available	Grows in lymph nodes
Leprosy	BCG → some protection	Immune spectrum: (lepromatous....tuberculoid)
Protozoa		
Malaria	Partial; antigenic variation Vaccines on trial	Immunosuppression; anaemia; nephritis
Trypanosomiasis		
African	Antigenic variation ++	Immunosuppression
Chagas'		Autoimmunity (CNS; heart)
Leishmaniasis	T cell dependent imm. Vaccines on trial	
Worms		
Schistosomiasis	Partial immunity Vaccines experimental	Egg-induced granuloma (liver, bladder)
Filariases	Little or no immunity	Immunopathology ++
Hydatid (tape) worm		Cyst rupture → anaphylaxis

Fig. 5 **Many of the world's most serious infections are essentially restricted to the tropics — often by the distribution of their vector.** Immunity is weak and may be absent and vaccines are mostly still experimental. DIC: disseminated intravascular coagulation.

Vaccination

The aim and the ideal

Vaccination, named after Jenner's cowpox vaccine for smallpox (1798) but nowadays applied to all forms of active immunization, aims to induce *memory* in T and/or B lymphocytes through the injection of a non-virulent antigen preparation. Thus the first actual infection is met by a secondary rather than a primary response; this may be against the microbe itself or against a toxin. The ideal vaccine would protect the individual and ultimately eliminate the disease (as happened with smallpox in 1980), but most vaccines simply protect the individual.

The antigen

In principle anything from whole organisms to small peptides can be used, but in practice most vaccines consist of either attenuated organisms, killed organisms, inactivated toxins or subcellular fragments (Fig. 1). Recently it has been shown that the genes for one or more antigens can be inserted into a living vaccine (usually virus) 'vector', and experiments are being done with totally synthetic peptides, the idiotype network, and even DNA itself.

When and who?

With some local variations, a more or less standard set of vaccines is now in use world-wide, some of which are (or should be) given to everyone and others only to those particularly at risk (Fig. 2). The timing of vaccination depends on the likelihood of infection, vaccines against common infections being given as early as possible allowing for the fact that some vaccines do not work properly in very young infants (Fig. 3).

Living versus non-living

There is a fundamental distinction between all live and all 'dead' vaccines (Fig. 4). Live ones consist of organisms (nearly always viruses) that have been *attenuated* by growth in unfavourable conditions, forcing them to mutate their genes; mutants that have lost virulence but retain antigenicity are repeatedly selected. Such organisms, which are essentially new strains, can sometimes regain virulence by back-mutation and can also cause severe disease in immunocompromised individuals. On the other hand they often induce stronger and better localized immunity and do not require 'booster' injections. Nowadays mutation is usually 'site-directed' by recombinant DNA technology. Killed organisms are used when for some reason stable attenuated ones cannot be produced. In only one case — polio — is there a choice between effective live and killed vaccines.

Passive immunization

In pre-antibiotic days, it was common to treat or prevent infection by injecting antibody preformed in another animal, usually a horse or a recently recovered patient. This principle is still in use for certain acute conditions where it is too late to induce active immunity by vaccinating the patient (Fig. 5). Gammaglobulin injections are also used for antibody deficiencies (see p. 53). Note that all blood products for injection must be screened for Hepatitis B and HIV.

Adjuvants

Non-living vaccines, especially those consisting of small molecules, are not very strong antigens but can be made stronger by injecting them along with some other substance such as aluminium hydroxide; such substances are called adjuvants. A variety of microbial, synthetic and endogenous preparations have adjuvant activity, but at present only aluminium salts are generally used (Fig. 6).

Type of antigen	Examples	
	Viruses	Bacteria
Normal heterologous organism	Vaccinia (cowpox)	
Living attenuated organism	Measles	BCG
	Mumps	Typhoid (new)
	Rubella	
	Polio: Sabin	
	Yellow fever	
	Varicella-zoster	
Whole killed organism	Rabies	Pertussis
	Polio: Salk	Typhoid
	Influenza	Cholera
Subcellular fragment Inactivated toxin (toxoid)		Diphtheria
		Tetanus
		Cholera (new)
Capsular polysaccharide		Meningococcus
		Pneumococcus
		Haemophilus
		Typhoid (new)
Surface antigen	Hepatitis B	

Fig. 1 Antigens in use as vaccines vary from whole living organisms to small molecules. New vaccines are being developed all the time; those shown in brackets are on trial but it is too soon to say they will become standard.

Recommendation	Vaccine	Regimen
All	Diphtheria	3 doses sc or im
	Tetanus	from 2–3
	Pertussis	dip/tet boost at 5 yr
	Measles	3 doses sc or im
	Mumps	from 1 yr (6/12 in tropics),
	Rubella	boost at 10–14 yr
	Polio (Sabin)	3 doses orally 2–6/12
	(or *Salk)	3 doses im
All, unless Mantoux +	BCG	i/d 10–14 yr (at birth in tropics)
At risk	Hepatitis B	3–4 doses im, 1–6/12 intervals
		(childhood in tropics)
		(at birth in Far East?)
	Hepatitis A	
	Influenza	Institutions, nurses, etc.
		Annual boost needed
	Rabies	Travel: 2–3 doses im
		Post-exposure: 5–6 doses plus
		antibody
	Meningococcus	Epidemics
	Pneumococcus	Elderly
	Haemophilus	Children
	Varicella-zoster	Leukaemic children
At risk (travel)	Typhoid	1 dose im
	Cholera	1 dose im
	Yellow fever	1 dose sc; boost 10 yearly

Fig. 2 The principal vaccines in use today. Note that regimens vary somewhat from country to country; usually this is because the disease in question is a bigger threat at a younger age in tropical areas.
* The Salk is the polio vaccine of choice in Holland and Scandinavia.

Vaccine	When given	Reason
Measles Mumps Rubella	1–1.5 yr	Maternal antibody
Pneumococcus Meningococcus	2 yr	Children under 2 respond poorly to polysaccharides
BCG	10–14 yr (UK)	Disease now rare

Fig. 3 Ideally all vaccines would be given soon after birth, but some are deliberately delayed, for various reasons.

	Living (attenuated)	Non-living
Immunity	Strong; localized	May be weak
	Usually appropriate type	May be inappropriate (e.g. antibody vs CMI)
	Usually good memory	Memory variable (poor with polysaccharides)
	May induce 'herd' immunity	
Boosting	Usually not required	Often required
Adjuvant	Not required	Usually required
Safety	Unsafe in immunocompromised, may revert to virulence	Usually safe if properly inactivated
Storage	Depends on 'cold chain'	Usually no problem
Side-effects	Egg hypersensitivity (some viruses)	Toxicity (e.g. pertussis?)

Fig. 4 Living and non-living vaccines differ in many important respects, notably safety and effectiveness.

Infection	Source of antiserum	Indications
Tetanus	Immune human; horse	Post-exposure (plus vaccine)
Diphtheria	Horse	Post-exposure
Gas gangrene	Horse	Post-exposure
Botulism	Horse	Post-exposure
Varicella-zoster	Immune human	Post-exposure in immunodeficient
Rabies	Immune human	Post-exposure (plus vaccine)
Hepatitis B	Immune human	Post-exposure, prophylaxis
Hepatitis A	Pooled human Ig	Prophylaxis
Measles	Immune human	Post-exposure in infants
Snakebite	Horse	Post-bite
Some autoimmune diseases	Pooled human Ig	Acute thrombocytopenia and neutropenia

Fig. 5 There are still a number of indications for passive immuni-zation by the injection of preformed antibody. Note that with repeated injections of horse antibody, there is the danger of immune complex formation and serum sickness. Antisera are usually injected intra-muscularly but can be given intravenously in extremely acute conditions.

In regular human use
Aluminium hydroxide
Aluminium phosphate
Calcium phosphate

Experimental, but likely to be approved
Liposomes[1]
MDP and derivatives[2]
ISCOM's[3]
Block co-polymers

Experimental only
Cytokines: IL-1, IL-2, IFNγ
Slow-release devices
Immune complexes

Fig. 6 Though a wide range of substances have been shown in experimental models to have adjuvant activity when given with vaccines, only aluminium and calcium salts are approved for general use in man. [1]Small synthetic lipid vesicles; [2]muramyl dipeptide, the postulated active component of mycobacterial cell walls; [3]immune-stimulating complexes, a lattice structure of the detergent Quil A.

Acquired Immunodeficiency Syndrome (AIDS)

AIDS was first reported in 1981 and has since resulted in the loss of at least half a million lives world-wide. AIDS is caused by infection with HIV-1. A related retrovirus HIV-2 causes a milder disease. It is estimated that more than 5 million people are currently infected with HIV-1. The HIV-1 virus is almost exclusively transmitted by body fluids. AIDS patients are defined as having persistent opportunistic infections (see p. 77) consistent with decreased cell-mediated immunity or tumours such as Kaposi's sarcoma and/or non-Hodgkin's lymphomas. Co-factors in the development of AIDS include genetic background but are commonly infections that repeatedly stimulate the immune system and facilitate the spread of HIV-1 in the patient's lymphoid organs. Avoidance of these co-factors seems to slow the progression of HIV infection.

Clinical spectrum of HIV infection

There is a spectrum of clinical symptoms during the progression of HIV-1 infection ranging from initial glandular fever-like symptoms in 10–20 % of patients, to persistent generalized lymphadenopathy, to full blown AIDS. The **AIDS-related complex (ARC)** is a clinical stage at which the patient has some symptoms of AIDS with at least two laboratory indications of reduced immune function, e.g. reduced CD4 T cell numbers and hypergammaglobulinaemia. The main immunological features of AIDS are shown in Figure 1. Following infection, some patients show no signs of immunodeficiency for 10 years or more, while others progress more rapidly.

Patients with AIDS die mainly from **opportunistic infections** (Fig. 2). The relationship between HIV and the development of *Kaposi's sarcoma* is unclear since HIV genes have not been found in Kaposi's cells. Other viruses may be involved, which emphasizes the importance of an intact immune system in resistance to virally induced tumours (see p. 85).

Serological responses to HIV

The development of antibody responses to HIV (seroconversion), as measured against the envelope glycoprotein gp120 and the core antigen p24, are shown in Figure 3. Screening of sera for HIV antibodies is carried out by ELISA and confirmed by Western blotting. Detection of the virus itself using molecular genetic techniques should also be carried out. Virus detection is important in neonatal diagnosis due to persistence of maternal antibodies. In utero infection may also be detected as IgM responses to the virus at birth.

Pathogenesis of AIDS

The receptor for HIV is CD4 expressed by T cells but also by macrophages and possibly very weakly by other cell types. The virus attaches via its gp120 envelope protein to CD4 on the surface of helper T cells (Fig. 4) and since the CD4 T cell plays a pivotal role in establishing immune responses it is not difficult to see how the virus weakens the entire immune system. The reason for CD4 T cell destruction is not totally clear since HIV is only weakly cytopathic and only a proportion of CD4 cells are infected. It is thought that secondary mechanisms play a role such as induction of apoptosis in CD4 T cells by gp120 viral proteins and cytotoxicity against CD4 T cells. Infection of macrophages leads to a decrease in IL-1 but increase in TNFα production. The increased levels of TNFα in AIDS patients are thought to contribute to both the **wasting disease** and **acute respiratory distress syndrome** (see p. 59) seen in some patients. HIV in macrophages is thought to represent a 'reservoir' of virus. As the disease progresses the absolute numbers of CD4 T cells decrease in the circulation whilst CD8 T cells are slightly increased (Fig. 5). These CD8 cells appear to be activated and seem to have a high turnover. CD4 and CD8 T cell numbers in blood are monitored by flow cytometry (see p. 92).

Prevention and treatment of AIDS

Figure 6 shows the main strategies for controlling AIDS. Traditional vaccination methods are hampered because the genes coding for envelope proteins are continuously mutating (see pp. 77–80). The main strategy at present is to use anti-viral treatment and combination therapy with reverse transcriptase inhibitors. Future immunological approaches are directed towards vaccine stimulation of T cell immunity, attempts to block viral entry and perhaps manipulation of the cytokine network. Blood products are now routinely screened for HIV.

Reduction in absolute blood CD4+ T cell counts
(used in monitoring progression of disease *)

Reduced delayed hypersensitivity responses

Decreased proliferation to soluble antigens

Decreased synthesis of IL-2 in vitro following
stimulation with antigens

Decreased mitogen response in vitro

Increased serum β2 microglobulin levels

Hyper- gammaglobulinaemia especially of IgA, IgG$_1$, IgG$_3$
and IgM

Moderate decrease in natural killer cell function

Fig. 1   Major immunological changes in AIDS.* The laboratory
diagnosis of AIDS is made when the patient has <200/mm^3 CD4 T
lymphocytes.

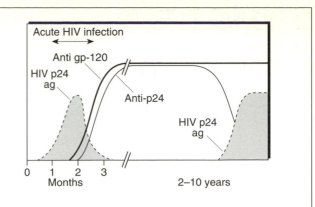

Fig. 3   Serological pattern of response following HIV infection.
p24 core antigen is detectable first. Antibodies to gp120 rise and
persist throughout the disease; levels of anti p24 rise as the levels of
antigen drop. Antibodies to another envelope protein gp41 are also
found (not shown).

Organisms	Main sites affected
Pneumocystis carinii (Europe & USA)	Lungs (pneumonia)
Cryptococcus	Lungs (pneumonia)
Mycobacteria	Lungs (pneumonia)
Tuberculosis (tropics)	
M. avium	
Toxoplasma gondii	Brain
Cryptococcus	Brain
Aspergillus	Brain
CMV	Brain, eyes, lungs
Candida	Mucosal surfaces

Fig. 2.   Main opportunistic infections seen in AIDS patients.

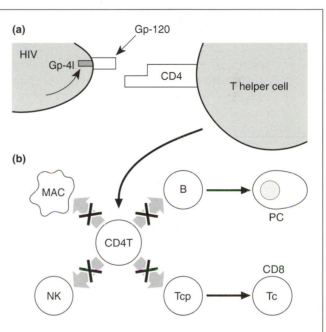

Fig. 4   HIV infection compromises the pivotal role of CD4 T cells.
Tcp, cytotoxic T cell precursor.

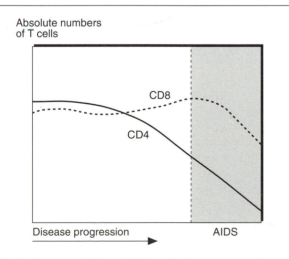

Fig. 5   Changes in CD4 and CD8 T cells after seroconversion.
This occurs at variable times after HIV seroconversion; levels of CD8
are usually higher after HIV infection than normal but at later stages
pan-lymphopenia can develop.

Strategy	Method
Virus neutralization	Vaccination — the search continues for a good vaccine
Blocking entry	Soluble CD4 (immunoadhesin)
	Anti-CD4 directed to virus-binding site
Inhibition of viral replication (HIV is a retrovirus)	Reverse transcriptase inhibitors: zidovudine (AZT), nucleoside analogues*

**Fig. 6   Strategies for prevention and treatment of AIDS. *May
be used in combination.**

Clinical Aspects of HLA

Genes of the HLA loci are highly polymorphic and in clinical medicine a patient's HLA type may need to be determined (1) to improve matching of foreign transplants (allografts) or (2) as an aid to diagnosis for a limited number of diseases, e.g. ankylosing spondylitis.

HLA and transplantation

The mechanisms of rejection have previously been described (see p. 51). In this section we will describe particular features of the important organ/tissue transplants.

- **Kidney.** The main indication for transplantation is end-stage chronic renal failure. The source of the transplant may be (1) living healthy relatives who are free of infection and malignancy or (2) cadavers which have been HLA *typed*. Both kinds of donors must also be ABO compatible and HLA *cross-matched* where possible. The three categories and causes of renal graft rejection are shown in Figure 1. Cyclosporin A, together with prednisone and azathioprine ('triple therapy') have improved the success rate of HLA-DR matched renal grafts at 5 years to around 80%. Even with two or more HLA-DR mismatches and the same triple therapy, the success rate is around 60%.
- **Liver.** Indications include hepatocellular carcinoma, biliary atresia, primary biliary cirrhosis, post-hepatic cirrhosis and alcoholic cirrhosis. Survival is currently 70% after 1 year and 60% at 5 years. Surprisingly there is no evidence that HLA matching improves graft survival!
- **Heart.** Indications include intractible heart failure and some rare congenital abnormalities. Triple therapy has increased survival to 80% at 4 years; the major cause of death is accelerated atherosclerosis in the coronary ateries of the graft in patients surviving beyond 1 year. Combined heart–lung transplants are becoming more common; success rates are low.
- **Bone marrow.** Indications for a bone marrow graft are given in Figure 2. Problems arise mainly from 'failure to take' of the graft, infections and HLA mismatching, the last giving rise to acute and/or chronic 'Graft versus host' (GVH) disease (Fig. 3). A mild GVH response from BM grafts is of value in treating some patients with tumours. GVH disease is avoided when autologous transplants are used for treatment of leukaemias but there is still the problem of residual tumour cells. The use of monoclonal antibodies to tumour-associated antigens to remove the tumour cells before grafting looks promising for the future (see p. 87, 88) .
- **Cornea.** There is no rejection unless the graft becomes vascularized, as occurs in about 5% of cases. Matching for regrafts is important due to sensitization by the first graft.
- **Skin.** Allografts of skin are used for short-term protection of patients with severe burns, being rejected within 2 weeks or so.
- **Pancreatic islet** and **parathyroid cells**. Transplantation is still experimental.

HLA and disease

The genes of the HLA system are grouped together on chromosome 6 and are usually inherited en bloc (see p. 51). Recombination between maternal and paternal chromosomes can occur but at low frequency (1%). Certain HLA alleles occur more frequently together than if there was a random assortment of individual alleles. This is termed **linkage disequilibrium** and is measured as the difference between the observed and statistically expected frequency of a particular combination of alleles. The reason for linkage disequilibrium is at present unclear but it may signify selective advantages of a given combination of alleles, for instance reduced susceptibility to a particular infection. However, the frequency of certain HLA alleles can also be higher in ('associated with') specific diseases. The association of a disease with a particular HLA allelic product (antigen) can be determined by calculating the **relative risk** (RR) (Fig. 4).

The archetypal HLA-association is that of ankylosing spondylitis with HLA-B27 where an individual with this HLA allele has around 90 times more chance of developing the disease than one without it. This is currently the *only* association which is useful as an aid to diagnosis. A reference list of HLA-disease associations is shown in Figure 5. Note that B27 is also associated with Reiter's syndrome; perhaps similarity between B27 and bacteria (*Klebsiella*) accounts for these associations ('antigenic mimicry'). In the case of B8 and DR3, more weakly associated with several autoimmune diseases, a general cytokine imbalance may be the link.

Type	Time scale	Cause
Hyperacute*	Minutes to hours	ABO mismatch: preformed circulating cytotoxic antibodies to MHC class I of donor
Acute	Few weeks to months	Associated with increase in both MHC class I and II and CD8 T cell infiltration
Chronic	Months to years	Thickening of GBM, interstitial fibrosis, perhaps due to persistent deposition of IC formed with antibodies and soluble graft antigens

Fig. 1 Rejection of renal grafts. *Less common with cross-matching; GBM, glomerular basement membrane; IC, immune complexes.

Acute GVH	Chronic GVH
< 4 weeks	> 100 days after transplantation: progression from acute or de novo
Affects mainly skin, liver and GI tract (graded according to severity)	Localized or general; clinical features: SS, SCL, PBC
T cell mediated	T cell and autoantibodies?

Fig. 3 A comparison of acute and chronic GVH disease. GI, gastrointestinal; SS, Sjögren's syndrome; SCL, systemic sclerosis; PBC, primary biliary cirrhosis.

$$\text{Relative risk (RR)} = \frac{p\text{ (with)} \times c\text{(without)}}{p\text{ (without)} \times c\text{(with)}}$$

where p (with)	=	No. patients with defined HLA type
c(without)	=	No. controls without defined HLA
p(without)	=	No. patients without defined HLA
c(with)	=	No. controls with defined HLA

Fig. 4 Calculation of relative risk (RR). This is the chance that an individual with the disease-associated HLA has of developing the particular disease compared with an individual lacking that HLA antigen.

Indication	Specific disease
Anaemia (see p. 75)	Aplastic (severe forms)
	Fanconi' s anaemia
Leukaemia (see p. 85)	Acute lymphoblastic
	Acute myeloid
	Chronic myeloid
Immunodeficiency (see p. 53)	Reticular dysgenesis
	Severe combined (SCID)
	Chronic granulomatous disease (CGD)
	Wiskott–Aldrich syndrome (WAS)
Inborn errors in metabolism	Gaucher's disease
	Hurler's disease
	Thalassaemia
	Osteopetrosis

Fig. 2 Indications for bone marrow grafting.

Disease	Associated HLA antigen			
	DR	B	C	A
Rheumatological				
Ankylosing spondylitis	–	27(90)	–	–
Juvenile ankylosing spondylitis	–	27(5)	–	–
Reiter's disease	–	27(33)	–	–
Adult RA	4(7)	–	–	–
Sjögren's syndrome	3(10)	8	–	–
SLE(caucasian)	2(3) 3(3)	–	–	–
Dermatological				
Psoriasis	–	–	w6(13)	–
Alopecia	–	12	–	–
Behçet's syndrome	–	5(3)	–	–
Pemphigus (AJ)	4(25)	–	–	–
(Caucasians)	–	–	–	10(3)
(Japanese)	–	–	–	10(6)
Gastrointestinal				
Ulcerative colitis	–	5	–	–
Atrophic gastritis	–	7	–	–
Haematochromatosis	–	14	–	–
Coeliac disease	3(11)	8(8)	–	–
CAH	3(14)	8(9)	–	–
Endocrine				
Addison's disease	3(6)	8	–	–
IDDM	3(5) 4(7)	8(10)	–	–
Graves' disease	3(4)	8(2)	–	–
Hashimoto's thyroiditis	5(3) 3(3)	–	–	–
Neurological				
Multiple sclerosis	2(5) 3(3)	7(2)	–	–
Myasthenia gravis (early onset, female)	–	8(13)	–	–
Narcolepsy	2(130)	–	–	–
Renal				
Goodpasture's syndrome	2(13)	–	–	–
Cancer				
Thyroid	3(3) 1(6)	–	–	–
Allergies				
Ragweed pollen	2(10)	–	–	–

Fig. 5 Major disease associations. The RR (where known) is shown in brackets; –, no association; AJ, Ashkenase Jews; CAH, chronic active hepatitis; IDDM, insulin-dependent diabetes mellitus.

Malignant Disease

Tumours of the immune system

Tumours of the immune system include both lymphoid and myeloid cell malignancies, with a combined incidence in the UK approaching 25 per 100 000. We will here deal with those immunological aspects of value in diagnosis.

Leukaemias are generally circulating haemopoietic tumour cells which may infiltrate organs; **lymphomas** are non-recirculating tumours which may have a 'leukaemic phase'. Leukaemias can be either acute or chronic. It is a reasonable approximation that acute lymphoid leukaemias derive from immature lymphoid precursors while chronic lymphoid leukaemias originate from mature lymphoid cells. Early classifications of leukaemias were made on the basis of their morphological appearance, e.g. FAB (French–American–British) and lymphomas on their histological appearance (Rappaport). More recent classifications (e.g. Kiel) have been based on their subset of origin (i.e. T or B lymphoid). These tumours are of **monoclonal** origin, i.e. they derive from single cells which continue to proliferate while 'arrested' during their development. Monoclonality can be documented by a number of methods (see p. 91). Chromosomal changes are seen in chronic granulocytic leukaemia (9;22 translocation referred to as Philadelphia chromosome) and acute promyelocytic leukaemia (15;17 translocation), etc. The so-called 'target cell' where the original malignant transformation takes place is apparently different in the various malignancies as indicated in Figure 1. There is further heterogeneity since a malignant clone may have several stages of differentiation. For example, although in its typical form, B cell CLL is a malignancy of small B lymphocytes, in a few cases such cells are capable of secreting sufficient antibody to be detectable as an electrophoretic 'spike' in the patient's serum (see your text on chemical pathology). **Myelomas** are tumours of terminally differentiated plasma cells. Large amounts of monoclonal antibodies of different IgG or IgA subclasses are detected as serum 'paraproteins'. Some plasma cell tumours produce heavy chains without accompanying light chains (heavy chain diseases).

Immunophenotyping or immunodiagnosis using antibodies to enzymes and differentiation antigens (see CD markers, p. 99) on/in normal lymphoid and myeloid cells is now used to aid diagnosis, prognosis and to determine the most appropriate treatment. Markers commonly used to investigate lymphoid maligancies are seen in Figure 2.

The cellular basis of **Hodgkin's disease** is at present unclear but it usually begins as lymphadenopathy with later involvement of the liver, spleen, bone marrow and lungs. It is characterized by large neoplastic ('**Reed–Sternberg**') cells with large nuclear inclusions. The cellular immune responses are particularly affected in these patients.

Tumour immunity

Evidence for a protective role for the immune system against tumours comes from studies showing an increased incidence of tumours in patients with immunodeficiency states and those receiving immunosuppressive therapy (Fig. 3 and pp. 51 & 87).

Tumour antigens. As for any microorganism, in order for the immune system to carry out its function it has to first recognize the tumour cells as foreign. Unfortunately, tumour cells are very similar antigenically to their normal counterparts to which the host is of course tolerant (see self/non-self, p. 21). There is little evidence for antigens exclusive to tumour cells (**tumour specific antigens**) in man although they have been described for some experimental animal tumours. However, these have mainly been defined by antibodies and it remains possible that self peptides altered by oncogenic viruses or viral peptides themselves (see below) could still be the target of weak T cell responses against tumours. A number of **tumour associated antigens** have been described which are useful in aiding diagnosis and monitoring tumour progression: these 'normal' cellular constituents are present during differentiation but while absent or barely detectable on mature cells, can be 'aberrantly' expressed by tumour cells (Fig. 4).

Viruses and tumours. a number of viruses have been associated with various tumours (Fig. 5). Vaccination with hepatitis B protects against liver tumours whilst EBV and Papilloma virus vaccination holds out promise for the future.

Immunotherapy. Cytotoxic mechanisms (cellular and humoral) are not normally effective in killing tumour cells but ways are being tried to enhance their activity (p. 87).

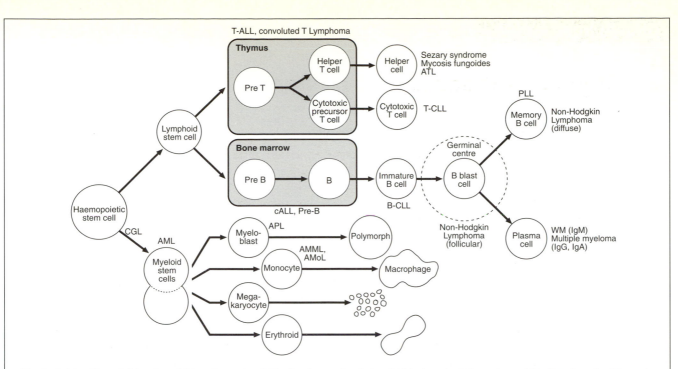

Fig. 1 Origin of lymphoid and myeloid malignancies. CGL, chronic granulocytic (myeloid) leukaemia; AML, acute myeloblastic leukaemia; APL, acute promyelocytic leukaemia; AMML, acute myelomonocytic leukaemia; AMoL, acute monocytic leukaemia; T–ALL, thymic acute lymphoblastic leukaemia; CALL, common acute lymphoblastic leukaemia; PRE–B, pre–B acute lymphoblastic leukemia; CLL, chronic lymphocytic leukaemia; PLL, prolymphocytic leukaemia; ATL, acute T cell lymphoma; WM, Waldenström's macroglobulinaemia.

Disease	Markers
Acute	
Common ALL	CD10,CD19,Mb-1(cyt), TdT(n)
'Null' ALL	CD19,Mb-1 (cyt), TdT (n)
Pre- B ALL	CD19,Mb-1 (cyt), IgM (m;cyt)
T ALL	CD7,CD3(cyt), TdT(n)
AML	CD13,CD33,myeloperoxidase (cyt)
AMML,AMoL	CD13,CD33,CD14,CD11c
CGL in blast crisis	
'Myeloid'	CD13,CD33,CD14,CD15
'Lymphoid'	TdT(n)
ATL	CD3,CD4
Chronic	
B-CLL	CD19,CD20,CD5,sIg+/±
HCL	CD19,CD20,TRAP
PLL	CD19,CD20,sIg++
Sezary/Mycosis Fungoides	CD3,CD4
T-CLL	CD3,CD8

Fig. 2 Markers used to help diagnosis of acute and chronic leukaemias. TdT, terminal deoxynucleotidyl transferase; (n), nuclear; Mb-1, a cytoplasmic Ig associated molecule (B-cell specific); (cyt), cytoplasmic; sIg, surface membrane immunoglobulin (+/++ refers to the intensity of expression); TRAP, tartrate resistant acid phosphatase.

Disease	Tumour type
Immunodeficiency	
Di George syndrome	
Wiskott–Aldrich syndrome	
Ataxia telangiectasia	All lymphoreticular
SCID	
Chediak–Higashi syndrome	
Immunosuppression	
Organ transplants -	
• azathioprine/steroids	NHL, liver cancer, Kaposi's sarcoma, cervical cancer
• cyclosporin A	Lymphoma, skin cancer, Kaposi's sarcoma
Inflammatory disease e.g. RA	NHL
Malaria	Burkitt's lymphoma
AIDS patients	NHL, Kaposi's sarcoma

Fig. 3 Increased incidence of tumours in immunodeficient and immunosuppressed patients. SCID, severe combined immunodeficiency; NHL, Non-Hodgkin's lymphoma; RA, rheumatoid arthritis. There is accumulating evidence that most of these tumours are caused by multiple factors including virally induced pathological changes (see Fig. 5).

Antigen	Distribution
Carcino-embryonic antigen (CEA)	Fetal gut cells: very small amounts on adult colonic cells but much higher on colonic tumour cells; antigen shed into serum aids diagnosis and progression
Alpha-fetoprotein	Secreted by fetal liver/yolk sac cells; serum of patients with liver or germinal cell tumours
cALL antigen (CD10)	Present on common acute lymphoblastic leukaemic cells; also on B lymphoid precursor cells in regenerating bone marrow or in fetal bone marrow

Fig. 4 Tumour-associated antigens.

Virus	Tumour	Co-factors
Epstein–Barr (EBV)	Burkitt's lymphoma, Nasopharyngeal carcinoma	Malaria Nitrosamines (in diet)
Hepatitis B	Liver cancer	Aflatoxin? (from moulds)
Papilloma virus	Cervical cancer Skin cancer?	
Human T cell leukaemia virus (HTLV-1)	T cell leukaemia (ATL)	

Fig. 5 Viruses associated with tumours and some possible cofactors for their development.

Drugs and the Immune System

Drugs used in immunological conditions

Immune responses can produce undesirable effects, such as allergy, autoimmunity and transplant rejection; the standard way to control these is by the use of **immunosuppressive** drugs. There are also certain circumstances in which drugs can be used to *stimulate* immunity.

Immunosuppression

In suppressing immunity, drugs can be targeted mainly at lymphocytes, or mainly at the macrophages and other cells of the natural immune system ('anti-inflammatory' drugs). Figure 1 lists the main drugs and their site of action. Note that their use is often limited by potentially serious side-effects, of which the most dangerous is the damage to dividing cells by cytotoxic agents such as azathioprine and cyclophosphamide. This affects not only lymphocytes but all proliferating cells, which of course includes the precursors of the platelets and granulocytes. Note also that suppression is generally 'across the board' rather than specific to the offending antigen (i.e. tolerance); the latter would be much more desirable but has proved difficult to achieve except in a few cases, such as desensitization to allergens.

Immunostimulation

The most successful form of immunostimulation is **vaccination**, which acts in an antigen-specific manner on lymphocytes (see p. 79). But various substances are used to non-specifically stimulate immune processes, including both endogenous molecules (e.g. cytokines) and foreign material (Fig. 2). This is a controversial area, but occasional dramatic results have been claimed in the treatment of infections and cancer with microbial or plant products, which may turn out to have an immunological basis.

Complications of drug therapy

In addition to the unwanted side-effects of immunosuppression mentioned above, some drugs can cause serious **hypersensitivity** reactions. Since most drugs are small molecules and not antigenic on their own, they usually need to bind to some protein or cell in order to stimulate an immune response; in immunological parlance they act as **haptens**. Hypersensitivity of all four classic Gell and Coombs' types can be induced in this way (Fig. 3). Unlike other adverse reactions to drugs, hypersensitivity occurs in an unpredictable and non-dose-dependent pattern but is unlikely to result from the first exposure to a drug. A few substances, however, can give symptoms similar to hypersensitivity on first exposure, for example, the **anaphylactoid** (anaphylaxis-like) reactions to radiological contrast materials which directly stimulate degranulation of mast cells.

Another unwanted effect of an immune response to a drug is that antibody against the drug may block its action; this can happen with cytokines and some hormones, and with antibodies themselves (e.g. mouse monoclonal antibodies used therapeutically against tumours, see Fig. 2).

Drug/indication	Activity	Main side-effects
Organ grafting		
Corticosteroids	Block IL-1, IL-6	Infection
Prednisone	Block migration	Hyperglycaemia
Prednisolone	Anti-inflammatory	Osteoporosis
Azathioprine	Blocks cell division, suppresses T cells	Infection, bone marrow suppression, neutropenia, thrombocytopenia
Cyclosporin	Blocks IL-2	Nephrotoxicity
FK 506	Blocks IL-2	
Anti-lymphocyte antibodies	Kill/block lymphocytes	Flu-like symptoms
Autoimmunity		
Corticosteroids	As above	As above
Azathioprine	As above	As above
Cyclosporin	As above	As above
Cyclophosphamide	Blocks cell division, suppresses antibody, inhibit PGs	Male sterility
NSAIDs		
Hypersensitivity		
Corticosteroids	As above	As above
Antihistamines	Block histamine	Sedation
Sodium cromoglycate	Stabilizes mast cells?	
Adrenaline	(For anaphylaxis)	

Fig. 1 **The major drugs used to inhibit undesirable immune responses.** NSAIDs, non-steroidal anti-inflammatory drugs (e.g. aspirin, indomethacin); PGs, prostaglandins.

Infection
Vaccines (specific)
Passive antibody
Adjuvants (non-specific)
Cytokines
Interferon α (for viral diseases)
Interferon γ (for CGD)
GCSF (to raise PMN count)

Tumours
Cytokines
Interferon α (for HCL)
IL-2 (for renal carcinoma)
Bacterial products
BCG
Streptococcal extracts, etc.
Antibody-toxin conjugates

Fig. 2 **The major agents used in attempts to enhance immunity.** CGD, chronic granulomatous disease, HCL, hairy cell leukaemia. For details of vaccines and adjuvants, see p. 79.

Gell and Coombs type and mechanism	Drugs	Clinical effect and comments
Type I; IgE, mast cells		
Allergic	Penicillin	Urticaria; angio-oedema
	Insulin	
Anaphylactic	Penicillin, cephalosporins, sulphonamides, foreign serum	75% of all anaphylaxis
Anaphylactoid	Contrast media, aspirin	
Type II		
IgG; cytotoxic	Penicillin	Haemolytic anaemia
	Quinidine	Haemolytic anaemia
	Methyldopa	Haemolytic anaemia (autoimmune)
	Quinidine, digoxin, sulphonamides	thrombocytopenic purpura
	Hydralazine, procainamide	Lupus syndrome (anti-DNA)
Type III		
Immune complex-mediated	Foreign serum	Serum sickness
Vasculitis	Thiazides	
	Sulphonamides, penicillin	
Type IV		
T cell mediated	Penicillin, cephalosporins	Contact dermatitis
'Delayed type'	Streptomycin, neomycin	
	Penicillin, sulphonamides, phenytoin, barbiturates, gold	Erythema multiforme, Stevens–Johnson syndrome, toxic epidermal necrolysis

Fig. 3 **The principal drugs causing hypersensitivity reactions, classified according to their immunological basis.** Note the importance of penicillin in all four major categories. Note also that not all 'drug reactions' are immunological.

Tutorial 5

You should now have a feeling for the role played by immune processes in a wide range of diseases. As before, test your knowledge by answering these questions.

Questions

1. What conditions favour the development of respiratory symptoms during an infection?

2. What immunological conditions of the digestive tract are often associated with disease elsewhere?

3. Which autoimmune endocrine conditions often occur together?

4. In what ways can antibodies damage the kidney?

5. What features of myasthenia gravis mark it as an autoimmune disease?

6. What important skin diseases have an immunological basis?

7. In a patient with signs of connective tissue disease, what is the value of detecting (a) rheumatoid factor, (b) anti-nuclear antibodies?

8. In what situations can a loss of red cells be due to antibodies?

9. What are the commonest opportunistic infections in immunodeficient patients?

10. Some vaccines are living and some are not. Why is this and what is the significance?

11. Distinguish between HIV infection, ARC and AIDS.

12. Why does an HLA mismatch not matter with (a) corneal and (b) liver grafts?

13. What common tumours arise from the B-cell lineage?

14. Which types of hypersensitivity can be triggered by penicillin?

Answers

1. Immunodeficiency (especially antibody deficiency; cystic fibrosis); organisms resistant to elimination (capsulated bacteria, fungi, mycobacteria); hypersensitivity reactions (e.g. allergies, granulomata); endotoxaemia (e.g. Gram-negative. bacteraemia leading to ARDS).

2. Sjögren's syndrome (eyes, mouth, joints, lymphoma); type A gastritis (pernicious anaemia and other autoimmunities); coeliac disease (dermatitis herpetiformis); Crohn's disease (eye); Wilson's disease (liver, brain, kidney); haemochromatosis (liver, pancreas, skin, etc).

3. Thyroid-pancreas (+ stomach, myasthenia gravis); adrenal–thyroid–pancreas–gonads; parathyroid–adrenal–gonads (+ candida, alopecia).

4. By leading to the formation of immune complexes that bind to glomerular endothelium or by directly binding to renal tissues. Examples of the latter are Goodpasture's syndrome (anti-basement antibodies affecting kidney and lung) and (rarely) antibodies against tubules. Examples of immune complex damage include infection (especially streptococci, hepatitis B, malaria, IgA nephropathy); systemic vasculitis (especially SLE); serum sickness.

5. The presence of autoantibodies to acetylcholine receptors in the blood and at the sites of damage on the muscle end-plate; the passive transfer of symptoms from mother to newborn; the beneficial effect of plasmapheresis; (suggestive only: the association with HLA B8 DR3 and with thymoma).

6. Allergic urticaria (type I hypersensitivity); angioneurotic oedema (C1 esterase inhibitor deficiency); the bullous diseases — pemphigus, pemphigoid, etc. (autoantibodies to skin components: type II); the vasculitides — SLE, Henoch–Schonlein, etc. (immune complexes: type III); allergic contact dermatitis (type IV). Some skin rashes (measles, typhoid) are due to the immune response, the pattern of some skin infections depending on the immune status of the patient (leprosy, leishmaniasis), and some skin conditions are predominantly seen in immunodeficient patients (muco-cutaneous candidiasis, Kaposi's sarcoma).

7. *Neither of these autoantibodies is diagnostic of anything.* However they can be useful in certain cases, as follows: rheumatoid factor is usually present in rheumatoid arthritis (70% of patients) but also in systemic sclerosis (30%); SLE (25%); absent in ankylosing spondylitis, Reiter's disease, infective arthritides. Anti-DNA antibodies are usually present in SLE (95%, mainly dsDNA), but also in drug-induced lupus, systemic sclerosis (c.60%), Sjögren's syndrome (60%), rheumatoid arthritis (30%).

8. Autoantibodies can cause haemolytic anaemia (warm type usually anti-Rhesus; cold type usually anti-blood group I). Antibodies to drugs can bind to red cells (e.g. penicillin). Antibodies to group A or B, or other blood groups in previously transfused patients, can cause a transfusion reaction. Maternal antibodies to fetal rhesus D antigen can cause haemolytic disease of the newborn. Antibodies to intrinsic factor (and possibly to gastric parietal cells) can cause pernicious anaemia. Rarely, anaemia may be caused by autoantibodies to erythroid precursors or to erythropoietin.

9. It depends on the nature of the immunodeficiency. Defects of myeloid cells, complement, antibody: mainly bacterial and fungal infections (e.g. staphylococci, *Strep. pneumoniae, Candida, aspergillus*, pneumocystis); C 5-9: *Neisseria*; T cell defects: viruses, intracellular bacteria, fungi, protozoa; AIDS: CMV, HSV, pneumocystis, mycobacterium (avium and tuberculosis), toxoplasma, histoplasma.

10. In general, living vaccines are more effective, but non-living ones are used when safe attenuation has not been achieved. Exceptions to this rule are: (a) subcellular fractions are effective against bacterial toxins (diphtheria, tetanus), bacterial capsules (*Strep. pneumoniae*, meningococcus, haemophilus) and HBV surface antigen; (b) living vaccines are not used in immunodeficient patients. In the special case of polio, living and killed vaccines are both in widespread use.

11. HIV infection, usually detected by testing for antibody, is the cause of AIDS (along with various undefined co-factors); however, some patients have remained symptom-free for 15 years or more, whilst others progress to AIDS within 2-3 years. ARC (AIDS-related complex) denotes a half-way stage, with at least two abnormalities (e.g. low CD4 T cells, an opportunist infection, hypergammaglobulinaemia). AIDS implies several major opportunist infections, and/or tumours (Kaposi's, lymphoma) and/or CNS changes (AIDS dementia).

12. With corneal grafts, there is normally no rejection because lymphocytes do not make contact with the graft and thus do not become sensitized to donor HLA. With liver grafts the explanation is probably that the grafted liver induces tolerance to HLA — either by virtue of its very large size, or perhaps by acting as a 'sump' for donor-specific host lymphocytes.

13. Acute lymphoblastic leukaemia (about 90% B, 10% T cell); chronic lymphocytic leukaemia (95% B); multiple myeloma; non-Hodgkin's lymphoma (mostly B, some T); *possibly* Hodgkin's disease. More rarely: hairy cell leukaemia; Waldenstrom's macroglobulinaemia; heavy chain disease.

14. All four main types. type I: urticaria, anaphylaxis; type II: haemolytic anaemia, neutropaenia; type III: interstitial nephritis, serum sickness; type IV: contact dermatitis, erythema multiforme. Of all these, anaphylaxis is the commonest and most dangerous.

Immunodeficiency/Tumours of the Immune System

Immunodeficiency

Tests for immune competence become necessary when: there is a history of congenital immunodeficiencies; infections are persistent and return after antibiotic treatment; patients have opportunistic infections; patients are treated with cytotoxic drugs or irradiation for cancer or prevention of graft rejection; patients receive a bone marrow graft for stem cell replacement.

Suspected phagocytic deficiencies:
- Quantitation of PMNs and monocytes from differential counts is undertaken in haematology.
- One measure of functional activity of PMNs is the nitroblue tetrazolium test (NBT: Fig. 1). More specialized tests include intracellular killing of bacteria by polymorphs.

Suspected complement deficiencies:
- Quantitation is accomplished using antibodies to the different components in gel diffusion.
- Functional complement activity can be measured using a haemolysis test.

Suspected antibody deficiencies:
- Quantitation of antibody classes by **gel diffusion** involves precipitation of serum immunoglobulins by antibodies to the various Ig classes in gels (see p. 23 and Fig. 2). Analysis is moving more towards nephelometry (measures precipitates in fluid phase) and ELISA (see p. 94). Note that normal serum values for immunoglobulins vary with age (see p. 100).
- Blood group isoagglutinins can be measured by **agglutination** techniques. Induced antibody responses can be measured following immunization with a vaccine, e.g. tetanus toxoid. (NB: Live vaccines should be avoided.)
- Absolute B lymphocyte numbers in the blood can be analysed using fluorescent antibodies and **flow cytometry** (see below).

Suspected T cell deficiencies:
- The analysis and counting of T lymphocytes is by a **fluorescent antibody technique** using monoclonal antibodies (see p.99). These reagents are labelled with different coloured fluorochromes and used in combinations. The laser-based **flow cytometer** measures the green or red fluorescence emitted by the individual antibody-labelled cells (see Figs 3a and 3b) as well as their morphology (i.e. size and granularity).
- Cell-mediated responses are measured in vivo by delayed hypersensitivity skin tests using a 'multitest' mixture of antigens including tuberculin and candida.

Tumours of the immune system

Lymphomas. T or B cell lymphomas can be distinguished in tissue sections using specific anti T cell (e.g. CD3) and anti B cell (e.g. CD20) antibodies labelled with fluorochromes (and examined by fluorescence microscopy) or enzymes (immunohistochemistry, using the same principle as the ELISA , see p. 94). Anti κ and λ light chain antibodies are used to analyse the monoclonal nature of B cell malignancies such as lymphomas and leukaemias as well as myelomas. The uniform gene rearrangement of Ig or TCR might be utilized to confirm these findings.

Lymphoid and myeloid leukaemias. These derive from different cell types and specific antibodies of the lymphohaemopoeitic system (see p. 85) and are distinguished by enzyme staining. These include CD13/CD33 for myeloid cells, CD3/CD5 for T cells and CD19/CD20 for B cells. An example for B-CLL is shown in Figure 3c and d. CD10 antigen is expressed on common acute lymphoblastic leukaemic cells (Figs 3e & 3f). Specific enzyme-linked antibodies to the various populations may also be used in blood smears. The cellular origin of these leukaemias determines treatment regimes and is related to prognosis.

Myelomas and other plasma cell tumours. Electrophoresis of both serum (Figs 4a & 4b) and urine (Figs 4c & 4d) can detect a variety of paraproteins including abnormal levels of different immunoglobulin classes, e.g. IgG (myelomas), IgM (Waldenström's macroglobulinaemia) and heavy or light chain diseases (see p. 85).

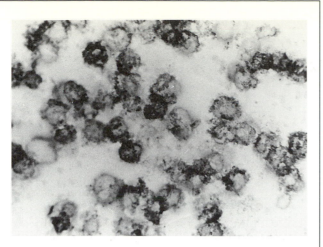

Fig. 1 **Nitroblue tetrazolium test (NBT).** Blue dye in healthy PMN indicates a normal respiratory burst.

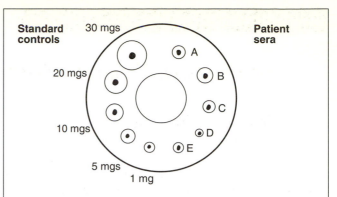

Fig. 2 **Measurement of serum immunoglobulins by gel diffusion.** Standard amounts of Ig are precipitated by class-specific antibodies in the agar gel. The diameter of precipitation is proportional to the Ig concentration and therefore the quantity of Ig in unknown sera (A–E) can be read off a calibration curve. These plates are commercially available.

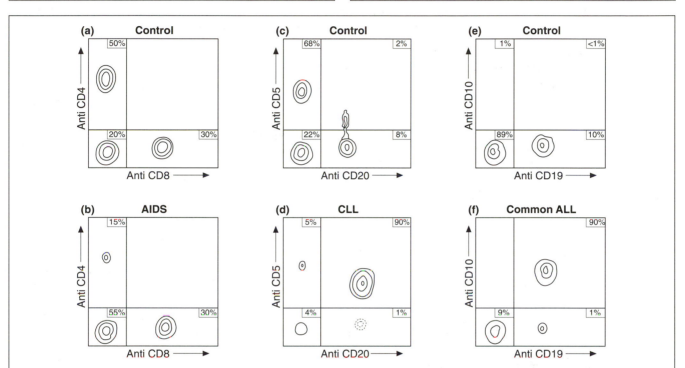

Fig. 3 **Analysis of lymphocyte populations by immunofluorescence and flow cytometry. (a)** Antibodies to CD4 (y-axis) and CD8 (x-axis) bind to blood lymphocytes and identify the two major distinct sub-populations of T cells. **(b)** Low numbers of CD4 T cells are detected In AIDS patient's blood. This gradual reduction in CD4 T cells is used to monitor the progression of disease. **(c)** Normal T cells are stained with anti CD5 antibodies (y-axis), whereas B cells are distinguished by their staining with anti CD20 antibodies (x-axis); a minor population of B cells also stains with CD5. **(d)** Most leukaemic cells from patients with B cell chronic lymphocytic leukaemia (CLL) express both CD5 and CD20. **(e)** In normal blood, no CD10 positive cells are seen but B cells (10%) are stained with anti CD19. **(f)** In common acute lymphoblastic leukemia (ALL) the blasts are CD10,CD19+ (B cell precursors). The residual cells (9%) are normal T cells (unlabelled).

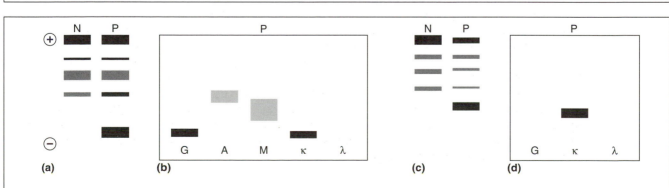

Fig. 4 **Identification of paraproteins by electrophoresis and immunofixation. (a)** Bands of proteins produced by electrophoresing serum in minigels show a large extra M band with the myeloma patient (P) compared with the control (N). **(b)** To identify the class of antibodies in the M band, strips of paper impregnated with different antibodies to the immunoglobulin classes are layered over the gel. Immunofixation of the M band occurs if antibodies bind to it. An IgGκ myeloma protein is shown. **(c)** The same technique can be applied to free light chains in the urine. **(d)** Note the κ Bence–Jones proteins in the urine of this patient with myeloma.

Allergy and Autoimmunity/The Transplant Patient

Investigating allergy

A careful history is often enough to establish the allergic origin of symptoms (seasonal or occupational), but the identification of the responsible antigen may require further clinical or laboratory testing.

- **Skin tests.** A *prick* test using a panel of likely allergens may reveal locally bound IgE. It is read after 10–20 minutes ('immediate hypersensitivity') and scored (e.g. 1+ to 4+) on the basis of wheal and erythema. An *intradermal* test is used for delayed hypersensitivity (e.g. the Mantoux test for TB); induration is read 2–3 days later. Contact sensitivity (e.g. to nickel) can be demonstrated by *patch* testing, read at 2 days.
- **Serum** can be assayed for total IgE (by immunoassay), for antigen-specific IgE (by RAST or MAST, see Fig. 1) or, in cases of suspected extrinsic allergic alveolitis, for antigen-specific IgG (by precipitin test, see Fig. 2).
- **Provocation tests** are sometimes used to identify the allergen responsible for hay fever or asthma. They are potentially dangerous and are only carried out by medical personnel in hospital.

Investigating autoimmunity

Autoantibody tests are an important part of the diagnosis of rheumatic diseases and some endocrine diseases. The ones most commonly requested are:

- **Rheumatoid factor**, in high titre, is virtually diagnostic of rheumatoid arthritis. The anti-Ig antibody is detected by agglutination of Latex particles or sheep red cells (Rose–Waaler test) coated with Ig.
- Antibodies to **double-stranded DNA** (for SLE), to the extractable nuclear antigens Sm (for SLE), Ro (SLE and Sjögren's syndrome) and La (Sjögren's), and to certain neutrophil enzymes (the ANCA test for various vasculitides). These are detected by radioimmunossay or ELISA (Fig. 3) if an initial screening by immunofluorescence (see below) is suggestive.
- Antibodies to uncharacterized **nuclear and cytoplasmic antigens**. These are detectable by indirect immunofluorescence on a range of tissues; the staining pattern is often sufficient to identify the site of binding, for example, with antinuclear antibodies (Fig. 4).

The transplant patient

Despite improvements in immunosuppression, **HLA typing** is still the keystone of successful organ transplantation, especially with bone marrow. This is a specialized test, only available in centres where transplants are carried out. There are several techniques in use:

- **Microcytoxicity** uses lymphocytes from the patient and monospecific typing sera (from multiparous women or, less often, post-transfusion) plus complement. Dead cells are read after 1 hour under phase-contrast. Class I antigens are detected by this method, but for Class II, purified B lymphocytes have to be used.
- **Cross-matching tests** involve the potential donor's cells being used as target in the above test, to detect pre-existing antibodies in the patient (e.g. due to transfusion or a previous transplant).
- **Lymphocyte-based tests**. The patient's T cells are typed by culturing with homozygous typing cells (HTC) irradiated to ensure that any resulting proliferative response is 'one way'. This should reveal all class II antigens capable of initiating a rejection response but has the disadvantage of taking 5–6 days. When there is a choice of donors (e.g. family members), the patient's and the donors' cells are set up as mixed lymphocyte cultures (MLC) in all combinations (Fig. 5).
- **Molecular biological methods** are the quickest and the most accurate of all. Examples are (1) restriction fragment length polymorphism (RFLP) plus Southern blotting and (2) the use of DNA probes combined with the polymerase chain reaction (PCR) to amplify individual DNA sequences (Fig. 6).

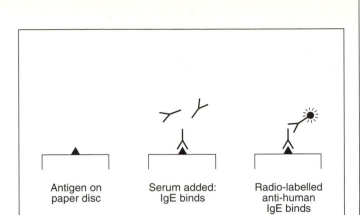

Antigen on paper disc | Serum added: IgE binds | Radio-labelled anti-human IgE binds

Fig. 1 The RAST (radio-allergo-sorbent) test is used to demonstrate serum IgE against a specific allergen. Up to 20 antigens can be tested at once. In a recent improvement (MAST), 35 antigens are banded on a single cellulose thread.

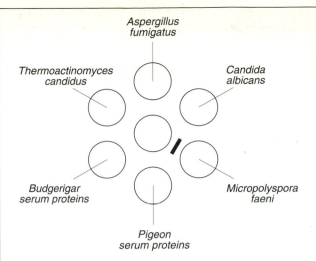

Aspergillus fumigatus

Thermoactinomyces candidus

Candida albicans

Budgerigar serum proteins

Micropolyspora faeni

Pigeon serum proteins

Fig. 2 A precipitin (Ouchterlony) test, showing the presence of specific IgG in a case of farmer's lung. The central well contains serum from the patient.

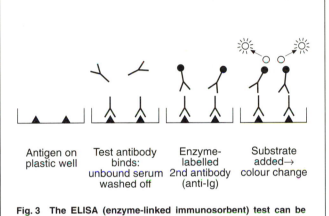

Antigen on plastic well | Test antibody binds: unbound serum washed off | Enzyme-labelled 2nd antibody (anti-Ig) | Substrate added→ colour change

Fig. 3 The ELISA (enzyme-linked immunosorbent) test can be used to demonstrate antibody against a known antigen, including some autoantigens.

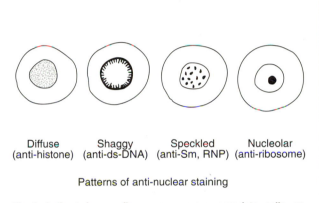

Diffuse (anti-histone) | Shaggy (anti-ds-DNA) | Speckled (anti-Sm, RNP) | Nucleolar (anti-ribosome)

Patterns of anti-nuclear staining

Fig. 4 Indirect immunofluorescence on appropriate cells or frozen sections can be used to demonstrate specific antibody in the serum.

Responder cells	Stimulator cells (irradiated)	DNA synthesis (c.p.m.)
Patient	Donor 1	8000
Patient	Donor 2	2500
Patient	[1]Patient	2000
Patient	[2]Unrelated	20000
Donor 1	Patient	9000
Donor 1	[1]Donor 1	4000
Donor 1	[2]Unrelated	30000
Donor 2	Patient	2000
Donor 2	[1]Donor 2	1500
Donor 2	[2]Unrelated	25000

Fig. 5 'Criss-cross' mixed lymphocyte culture. It is shown that Donor 2 would be the most suitable for the patient because there is less stimulation. Note the 'low' ([1]) and 'high' ([2]) controls.

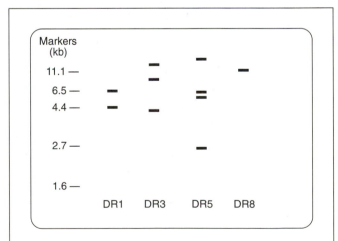

Markers (kb)

11.1 —
6.5 —
4.4 —
2.7 —
1.6 —

DR1 DR3 DR5 DR8

Fig. 6 Southern blot. In this test DNA from 4 homozygous patients has been digested with the restriction endonuclease Taq-I, run in gel electrophoresis and hybridized with a DNA probe giving characteristic patterns with different DR types. In a heterozygous patient, a mixture of two patterns will be seen.

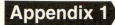

The Language of Immunology

Immunologists use a lot of jargon which can make a complicated subject even harder to get to grips with. Here are some words that crop up frequently and are either unique to immunology or are used in a special sense by immunologists.

Active/passive immunization: Protection against microbes is active when the immune system participates in the immune response (e.g. following vaccination) or passive when 'preformed' antibodies made in another individual or animal are injected.

Adhesion molecule: A cell surface molecule involved in cell–cell interactions.

Adjuvant: A substance which non-specifically potentiates an immune response to an antigen given with it (e.g. alum in human vaccines).

Affinity: The binding strength (association constant, K) between an individual ligand and receptor (e.g. one antibody binding site and one antigenic determinant).

Allograft: A tissue transplant between genetically different individuals within the same species.

Allotype: The protein product of an allele which may be detectable as foreign by another member of the same species (e.g. blood groups, MHC antigens or the allotypes on Ig).

Anergy: A potentially reversible state of tolerance which involves non-responsiveness rather than cell deletion.

Antigen: Strictly speaking, a substance that induces an antibody response, but generally used for any molecule that binds specifically to antibody or T cell receptors.

Antigenic determinant (see also epitope): The small portion of an antigen that is recognized and bound by antibody or the T cell receptor, usually about 9–20 amino acids in size. Thus even the smallest antigen will carry numerous determinants.

Apoptosis (programmed cell death): A mode of cell death which occurs under physiological conditions and is controlled by the dying cell itself ('cell suicide').

Atopy; atopic: IgE-mediated hypersensitivity or the tendency to develop this; more or less synonymous with allergy.

Autologous: Derived from the same individual.

Avidity (functional affinity): The binding strength between two molecules such as an antibody and an antigen. Avidity differs from affinity because it incorporates the valency of the antigen–antibody interaction: thus IgG has 2 binding sites and IgM has 10.

Carrier: An immunogenic molecule containing epitopes recognized by T cells (usually a protein). When a carrier is conjugated to a non-immunogenic hapten molecule it renders the hapten immunogenic.

Chemotaxis: Directional movement of cells in response to a concentration gradient of chemotactic factors such as bacterial peptides or cytokines.

Chimera: An animal or tissue composed of elements derived from genetically distinct individuals.

Class switching: The process by which B cells can express a new heavy chain isotype without altering the specificity of the antibody produced. This occurs by gene rearrangement.

Clonal selection: Selection of antigen-specific B or T cells by antigen and expansion into a clone. Burnet's clonal selection theory of 1959 was the first suggestion that this was how the antibody response worked.

Complex: (or 'immune complex'): The product of antigen and antibody, non-covalently bound in various proportions.

Conjugate: The product of covalent binding of two molecules, e.g. a toxin or a fluorescent molecule chemically bound to an antibody.

Cytophilic: Able to bind to cells, e.g. IgG antibodies through Fc receptors.

Cytotoxic: Able to kill cells — often referred to as the 'target'.

Domain: The structural unit into which the immunoglobulin heavy and light chains and members of the immunoglobulin gene superfamily are organized. Each unit consists of about 110 amino acids with an intrachain disulphide loop of about 60 amino acids that is folded into a three-dimensional structure known as the immunoglobulin fold.

Effector cells: Cells capable of mediating an immune function such as cell-mediated cytotoxicity, often used to contrast them with memory cells.

Epitope: The antigenic determinant or small part of an antigen site which interacts with an antibody or T-cell receptor.

Flow cytometry: Used to measure the phenotype and morphological characteristics of cell populations in suspension.

Germ line: The germ cells through which the continuity of the species is maintained; the term is used for those Ig genes inherited from the parents rather than generated by somatic mutation.

Hapten: A small molecule which is not immunogenic by itself but which, when coupled to a larger carrier molecule, can elicit antibodies directed against the hapten, e.g. some drugs.

Humoral: Refers to extracellular fluid, including the plasma and lymph. 'Humoral immunity' essentially means antibody-mediated immunity.

Hybridoma: An 'immortal' cell line derived by fusion of a T or B lymphocyte with a tumour cell, useful for making monoclonal antibodies (q.v.).

Hypervariable regions: Amino acid sequences within the variable regions of heavy and light immunoglobulin chains and of the T-cell receptor which show the most variability and contribute most to the antigen-binding site. Synonymous with complementarity determining regions (CDRs).

Idiotype: Set of individual antigenic determinants (idiotopes) of an immunoglobulin or T-cell receptor variable region, against which other ('anti-idiotypic') B or T cells can react.

Immunogen: A substance capable of eliciting an immune response. All immunogens are antigens; but some antigens, such as haptens, are not immunogens. Sometimes also used to describe antigens which induce actual protective immunity, e.g. against infection.

Integrins: One of the 'families' of adhesion molecules.

Isotype: Antibody class (IgM, IgG, IgA, IgD and IgE). Each isotype is encoded by a separate immunoglobulin constant region gene sequence that is carried by all members of a species (c.f. allotype).

Lectins: Proteins, usually derived from plants, which specifically bind sugars and oligosaccharides present on the membrane glycoproteins of animal cells.

Ligand: A molecule recognized by a given receptor (i.e. used in the same sense as in biochemistry).

Mimicry: The mechanism by which microbes avoid the immune response by having antigens similar to self-antigens to which the host is tolerant.

Mitogen: Any substance that non-specifically induces DNA synthesis and cell division (e.g. PHA).

Monoclonal antibodies: Antibodies produced by a cell clone and therefore identical with regard to specificity; used as standard laboratory reagents, e.g. for identification of cell surface markers, bacterial typing, etc.

Network theory: Theory proposing that the immune system is regulated by a network of idiotype and anti-idiotype reactions involving antibodies and T-cell receptors, put forward by Neils Jerne in 1974.

Null (cell): An out-of-date term for lymphocytes expressing neither T nor B cell markers.

Opportunist: A normally harmless microbe which results in serious infection only when the immune system is compromised (e.g. by HIV or a drug).

Opsonin: A substance, such as antibody or C3b, which binds to an antigen and enhances its phagocytosis, a process called opsonization.

Paratope: An idiotope or antigenic site on an antibody or T-cell receptor involved in binding to the epitope of an antigen.

Polyclonal: Involving many different clones of lymphocytes or antibodies secreted by several clones of lymphocytes.

Polymorphism: Presence of several alleles at a single gene locus (e.g. blood groups, the MHC).

Private/public: Idiotypes which are restricted to one individual are termed private whereas those idiotypes which are common within a species or between species are called public (or cross-reactive) idiotypes.

Prozone: The unexpected absence of a detectable reaction (e.g. immune precipitation or agglutination) at high concentrations of antibody.

Reagin: Often used to describe IgE antibodies.

Sensitization: The process whereby the adaptive immune system encounters antigen for the first time resulting in the development of memory.

Superantigens: Antigens (often bacterial) which bind to the MHC outside the peptide-binding groove and stimulate all or most of the T-cells bearing particular T-cell receptor V regions.

Syngeneic: Genetically identical members of same species, e.g. human identical twins or mice from an inbred strain.

Thy-I: One of the first glycoproteins to be found on the surface of most thymocytes and peripheral T cells.

Titre: The relative strength of an antiserum. It is the reciprocal of the last dilution of an antiserum capable of mediating some measurable effect such as precipitation or agglutination.

Tolerogen: Substance which induces a state of immunological tolerance.

Toxoid: Toxin that has been altered to eliminate its toxicity but retains its immunogenicity.

Transformation: Morphological changes in a lymphocyte associated with the onset of division. Also used to denote the change to the autonomously dividing state of a cancer cell.

Transgenic: An animal (usually a mouse) in which a foreign gene has been inserted to study its effect when expressed in a special site or manner.

Western blotting: Technique for identification of antigens in a mixture by electrophoresis, blotting onto nitrocellulose and labelling with enzyme or radiolabelled antibodies.

Xenograft: A graft between individuals of different species, e.g. a pig heart in man.

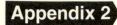

Some Useful Abbreviations

Immunologists are fond of abbreviations. The following are quite likely to turn up in lectures or discussion.

ADA	adenosine deaminase (e.g. deficiency)
ADCC	antibody-dependent cell-mediated cytotoxicity
AIDS	acquired immune deficiency syndrome
ALL/AML	acute lymphoblastic/myeloid leukaemia
ANA/ANF	Anti-nuclear antibody/factor
ANCA	anti-neutrophil cytoplasmic antibody
APC	antigen-presenting cell
ARC	AIDS-related complex
ARDS	adult respiratory distress syndrome
AS	ankylosing spondylitis
B cell	bursa (or bone marrow) derived lymphocyte
BCG	Bacille Calmette–Guerin (the TB vaccine)
BCGF/BCDF	B cell growth/differentiation factor(s) (now given IL numbers)
BETA 2 (M)	β_2 microglobulin
C	complement component (e.g. 1–9)
C	constant (genes, domains of Ig)
CD	cluster of differentiation (see Appendix 3)
CDR	complementarity determining region (e.g. of an antibody molecule)
CGD	chronic granulomatous disease
CLL/CML	chronic lymphocytic/myeloid leukaemia
CMI	cell (i.e. T cell)-mediated immunity
CMV	cytomegalovirus
CR	complement receptor
CRP	C-reactive protein
CREST (syndrome)	Calcinosis–Raynaud's–esophageal dysmotility–sclerodactyly-telangectasia
CSF	colony stimulating factor
CTL	cytotoxic T lymphocyte
D	diversity (genes/segments in Ig)
DTH	delayed-type hypersensitivity (often used as synonymous with cell-mediated immunity)
DPT	diphtheria–pertussis–tetanus (vaccine)
EBV	Epstein–Barr virus
ELISA	enzyme-linked immunosorbent assay
ENL	erythema nodosum leprosum
ESR	erythrocyte sedimentation rate
F(ab)	antigen-binding fragment (of Ig)
FACS	fluorescence-activated cell sorter
Fc	crystallisable (=constant) fragment of Ig
FcR	receptor for Fc
GVH(D)	graft-versus-host (disease; reaction)
H	heavy (chain of Ig molecule)
HBs (antigen)	hepatitis B surface antigen
HDN	haemolytic disease of the newborn
HEV	high endothelial venule (through which lymphocytes migrate)
HIV	human immunodeficiency virus
HLA	Human leukocyte antigen(s) — the human MHC antigens (and genes)
HSV	herpes simplex virus (types 1 and 2)
HTC	homozygous typing cell
HTLV	human T cell leukaemia virus
ICAM	intercellular adhesion molecule

Id	idiotype (e.g. of antibody molecule)	MIF	macrophage migration inhibitory factor (the first described cytokine)
IDDM	insulin-dependent diabetes mellitus	MLC/MLR	mixed lymphocyte culture/reaction
IF	immunofluorescence	NBT	nitroblue tetrazolium (assay)
IFN	interferon	NHL	non-Hodgkin's lymphoma
Ig	immunoglobulin	NK cell	natural killer cell
IL	interleukin	PAF	platelet-activating factor.
ISCOM	immune stimulating complex (a type of synthetic adjuvant)	PALS	periarteriolar lymphoid sheath
J	joining (genes/segments of Ig or TCR)	PCA	passive cutaneous anaphylaxis
		PCR	polymerase chain reaction
J	joining (chain of IgA molecule)	PG	prostaglandin
JRA	juvenile rheumatoid arthritis	PHA	phytohaemagglutinin (sometimes used as a polyclonal T cell stimulant)
K cell	'killer' cell (a somewhat outdated term for the cell(s) involved in ADCC)	PMN	polymorphonuclear leucocyte (also known as neutrophil)
L	light (chain of Ig molecule)	PPD	purified protein derivative (of *M. tuberculosis*, used for skin testing)
LAK cell	lymphokine-activated killer cell (an experimental strategy for treating cancer)	RA	Rheumatoid arthritis
LFA	lymphocyte function antigen (used for some cell adhesion molecules).	RAST	radio-allergo-sorbent test (for IgE)
		RES	reticulo-endothelial system
		RIA	radio immunoassay
LGL	large granular lymphocyte	SCID	severe combined immunodeficiency
LPS	lipopolysaccharide (endotoxin)	SLE	systemic lupus erythematosus
LT	lymphotoxin (also known as TNFβ)	T cell	thymus-derived lymphocyte
MAC	membrane attack complex (of complement)	T_C/T_H	cytotoxic/helper T cell
		TCGF	T cell growth factor (now IL-2)
MAC	often used as short for macrophage	TCR	T cell receptor
MAF	macrophage-activating factor (e.g. IFNγ)	TGF	transforming growth factor
		TNF	tumour necrosis factor (often applied particularly to TNFα)
MALT	mucosa-associated lymphoid tissue	TSH	thyroid stimulating hormone
MAST	multiple allergo-sorbent (or allergy screening) test	TSTA	tumour-specific transplantation antigen
M(C)Ab	monoclonal antibody	V	variable (genes/region of Ig or TCR)
MHC	major histocompatibility complex (in humans: HLA)	VZV	varicella-zoster virus

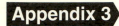

Cluster of Differentiation Antigens

Antigen	Other names/functions	Ligand	Cell distribution
CD 1a			Thy, DC, LHC
1b			Thy, LHC
1c			Thy, DC, B sub
2	SE-receptor	CD58	T, NK sub
2R			T act
3		Ag/MHC	All T cells
4		MHC II HIV-1,2	T sub
5		CD72	T, B sub;
6			T sub, B sub
7			T sub, NK and Pt
8		MHC I	T sub
9			Pre-B.M.Pt
10	CALLA, neutral endopeptidase	Peptides	Pre-B,G
11a	LFA-1α	CD54 ICAM-2	Leukocytes
11b	MAC-1, CR-3	C3bi, FIB	M, G, NK
11c	CR-4	C3bi	M,G, NK, B sub
w12			M,G,Pt
13	aminopeptidase N	Peptides	M.G
14		LPS binding Protein	M, G, LHC
15	X-hapten, Le^x	CD62	G.M
16	Fcγ RIII	Fc (IgG)	NK, G, M sub
w17	lactosylceramide		G, M, Pt
18	Integrin β2-chain β chain of CDIIa,b,c	CD54 ICAM-2	Leukocytes
19			B
20	? ion channel		B
21	CR2	C3bi.EBV	B, FDC
22		ME	B cells (resting ?)
23	Fcε RII	Fc (IgE) lo	B, B act, M act, Eo
24			B, G
25	IL-2 Rα, Tac	IL-2	T act, B act, M act
26	dipeptidyl peptidase IV	peptides	T act, B act, Mac
27			T sub
28		B7(CD80)	T sub, B act
29	VLA, integrin β1-chain	FN, collagen VCAM-1	Broad
30			T act, B act, RS
31	PECAM-1		Pt, M, G, B
32	FcγRII	Fc (IgG)	Mac, G, B, Eo
33			M, BM
34			BM
35	CR1	C3b	G, M, B, NK sub, RBC
36	Pt-GPIV	Thrombo-spondin	M, P
37			B
38			PC, T act, Thy
39			B, FDC, M
40		T cell gp39	B, FDC
41	Pt-GPIIb, integrin αIIb	FIB, FN, VN, vWF	Pt

Antigen	Other names/functions	Ligand	Cell distribution
42a	Pt-GPIX	vWF	Pt
CD 42b	Pt-GpIb	vWF	Pt
43	Leukosialin	?CD54	T, G, M
44	Pgp-1, ECMR-III	Hyaluronate	Leukocytes, RBC
45	LCA, PTPase	Tyr-P	Leukocytes
45RA	Restricted LCA	Tyr-P	T sub, B, M,
45RB	Restricted LCA	Tyr-P	Leukocytes
45RO	Restricted LCA	Tyr-P	T sub, B sub, G, M
46	MCP		Leukocytes, Pt
47			Broad
48			Leukocytes
49a	VLA-α1	lam, coll	Broad
49b	VLA-α2.Pt-GPIa	coll	Leukocytes, Pt
49c	VLA-α3	FN, lam, coll	Broad
49d	VLA-α4	VCAM-1	M, B, T, Thy, Pt
49e	VLA-α5, FNRα	FN	Broad
49f	VLA-α6	lam	Pt.
50	ICAM-3		Leukocytes
51	VNR α chain	VN	Pt. leukocytes
52	Campath-I		Leukocytes
53			Leukocytes, BM
54	I-CAM 1	CDIIa/18 rhinovirus	Broad
55	DAF		Broad
56	N-CAM, NKH1	CD56	NK, T sub
57	NHK1		NK, T sub,
58	LFA-3	CD2	Broad
59	TAP, Protectin		Broad
w60	GD3		T sub, Pt
61	Pt-GPIIIa, VNRβchain	VN, FN, FIB	Pt
	β-3 integrin chain	v W F	
62E	ELAM-I, E-Selectin		End act
62L	LAM-1, L-Selectin		T sub, B sub
62P	P-Selectin	CD15	Pt act, end act
63			Pt, M
64	FcγRI	Fc (IgG)	M, Mac
w65	Ceramide Dodecasaccharide 4c		G, M
66			G
67			G
68			Mac
69			Mac, act T/B/NK
70		CD27	T act; B act, RS
71	Transferrin receptor	transferrin	Mac, prolif cells
72	Lyb-2	CD5	B
73	Ecto-5′-nucleotidase	NMP	B sub, T sub
74	MHC II invariant chain		B, M
75	α2,6 sialyltransferase		B, T sub
w76			B, T sub
77	Gb3, Globotriasyl Ceramide		B
w78			B
79a	MB1, Igα chain		B
79b	B29, Igβ chain		B
80	B7, BB1	CD28	B, Mac
89	FcαR	Fc (IgA)	M, Mac, G

CD (cluster of differentiation) antigens are defined by groups of monoclonal antibodies which recognize leukocyte-derived molecules with a common molecular mass and cellular distribution. A series of workshops are organized frequently to define different CDs. Those antigens currently being characterized by a workshop are prefixed by w. Note: this list is constantly being added to, particularly as cytokine receptors become characterized. Abbreviations: **Thy**, thymocytes; **DC**, dendritic cells; **LHC**, Langerhans cell; **T**, T cell; **B**, B cell; **Pre-B**, pre-B cell; **G**, granulocyte; **M**, monocyte; **Mac**, macrophage; **Eo**, eosinophil; **BM**, bone marrow cell; **sub**, subset; **SE**, sheep erythrocyte; **NK**, natural killer cell; **act**, activated; **MHC**, major histocompatibility complex; **End**, endothelial cells; **HIV**, human immuno-deficiency virus; **Pt**, Platelet; **CR**, complement receptor; **ME**, mouse erythrocyte receptor; **LCA**, leukocyte common antigen; **LPS**, lipopolysaccharide; **Tyr-P**, tyrosine phosphatase; **VN**, vitronectin; **VNR**, vitronectin receptor; **FIB**, fibrinogen; **FN**, fibronectin; **FNR**, fibronectin receptor; coll, collagen; **lam**, laminin; **MCP**, membrane cofactor protein; **DAF**, decay accelerating factor; **VCAM**, vascular cell adhesion molecule; **ICAM**, intercellular adhesion molecule; **vWF**, von Willebrand factor; **RS**, Reed-Sternberg cell; **PC**, plasma cell.

Changes in Circulating Lymphocyte Populations and Serum Immunoglobulin Levels with Age

Cells		Cord blood	1 day–11 months	1–6 years	7–17 years	18–70 years
Lymphs*(%)		41 (35–47)	47 (39–59)	46 (38–53)	40 (36–43)	32 (28–39)
	(**Abs)	5.4 (4.2–6.9)	4.1 (2.7–5.4)	3.6 (2.9–5.1)	2.4 (2.0–2.7)	2.1 (1.6–2.4)
T	(%)	55 (49–62)	64 (58–67)	64 (62–69)	70 (66–76)	72 (67–76)
	(Abs)	3.1 (2.4–3.7)	2.5 (1.7–3.6)	2.5 (1.8–3.0)	1.8 (1.4–2.0)	1.4 (1.1–1.7)
CD4+	(%)	35 (28–42)	41 (38–50)	37 (30–40)	37 (33–41)	42 (38–46)
	(Abs)	1.9 (1.5–2.4)	2.2 (1.7–2.8)	1.6 (1.0–1.8)	0.8 (0.7–1.1)	0.8 (0.7–1.1)
CD8+	(%)	29 (26–33)	21 (18–25)	29 (25–32)	30 (27–35)	35 (31–40)
	(Abs)	1.5 (1.2–2.0)	0.9 (0.8–1.2)	0.9 (0.8–1.5)	0.8 (0.6–0.9)	0.7 (0.5–0.9)
CD4:CD8		1.2 (0.8–1.8)	1.9 (1.5–2.9)	1.3 (1.0–1.6)	1.3 (1.1–1.4)	1.2 (1.0–1.5)
B	(%)	20 (14–23)	23 (19–31)	24 (21–28)	16 (12–22)	13 (11–16)
	(Abs)	1.0 (0.7–1.5)	0.9 (0.5–1.5)	0.9 (0.7–1.3)	0.4 (0.3–0.5)	0.3 (0.2–0.4)
NK	(%)	20 (14–30)	11 (8–17)	11 (8–15)	12 (9–16)	14 (10–19)
	(Abs)	0.9 (0.8–1.8)	0.5 (0.3–0.7)	0.4 (0.2–0.6)	0.3 (0.2–0.3)	0.3 (0.2–0.4)

Changes in lymphocyte populations in the circulation as a function of age: values are given as medians with percentiles p25–p75 since distributions of many lymphocyte populations are asymetrical. *Lymphocytes expressed as a percentage of the total white blood cell count (WBC). **Absolute counts are expressed in 10^3 cells per mm^{-3}: T cells are defined as CD3+ lymphocytes, B cells as CD19/CD20+ and NK cells as CD3–/CD16+, CD56+ cells. Note a general decrease in lymphocyte numbers with age. (Modified from Hannet I, Erkeller–Yuksel F, Lydyard P M, De Bruyere M 1992 *Immunology Today*, Vol 13: p. 215).

Age		IgM g/L	IgG g/L	IgA g/L
Cord		0.02–0.2	5.2–18.0	< 0.0.2
Weeks	0–2	0.05–0.2	5.0–17.0	0.01–0.08
	2–6	0.08–0.4	3.9–13.0	0.02–0.15
	6–12	0.15–0.7	2.1–7.7	0.05–0.4
Months	3–6	0.2–1.0	2.4–8.8	0.10–0.5
	6–9	0.4–1.6	3.0–9.0	0.15–0.7
	9–12	0.6–2.1	3.0–10.9	0.20–0.7
Years	1–2	0.5–2.2	3.1–13.8	0.3–1.2
	2–3	0.5–2.2	3.7–15.8	0.3–1.3
	3–6	0.5–2.0	4.9–16.1	0.4–2.0
	6–9	0.5–1.8	5.4–16.1	0.5–2.4
	9–12	0.5–1.8	5.4–16.1	0.7–2.5
	12–15	0.5–1.9	5.4–16.1	0.8–2.8
	15–45	0.5–1.9	5.4–16.1	0.8–2.8
	> 45	0.5–2.0	5.3–16.5	0.8–4.0

Normal ranges for immunoglobulin levels in UK Caucasians: these are expressed as 5th–95th centile ranges. Note that adult levels of IgM are reached by about 1 year of age. IgG levels, high at birth since they are maternal antibodies transmitted across the placenta, decrease up to about 9–12 months and then increase as de novo IgG becomes apparent (see pp. 23–24). IgA levels continue to increase throughout life.

Index